Meal Prep Cookbook

200 Easy to Make Healthy Meal Prep Recipes for Weight Loss and Peak Health

Gregory Moore

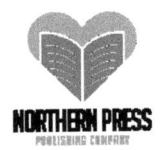

NORTHERN PRESS
PUBLISHING COMPANY

Copyright © by Northern Press

All rights Reserved. This book or any portion thereof may not be reproduced or used in any manner whatsoever without the express written permission of the publisher except for the use of brief quotation in a book review. The scanning, uploading, and distribution of this book via the Internet or via any other means without the permission of the publisher is illegal and punishable by law.

Please purchase only authorized editions of this book and don't participate in or encourage electronic piracy of copyrighted materials.

If you would like to share this book with another person, please purchase an additional copy for each person you share it with, or ask them to buy their own recipes. This was hard work for the author and he appreciates it.

This book is solely for information and education purposes and is not medical advice. Please consult a medical or health professional before you begin any exercise, nutrition, or supplementation program or if you have questions about your health.

Specific results mentioned in this book should be considered extraordinary and there are no "typical" results. As individuals differ, then results will differ.

Published by Northern Press Inc.

BREAKFAST RECIPES	10
GREEN PINA COLADA SMOOTHIE	11
CHOCOLATE SMOOTHIE	11
PROTEIN SMOOTHIE	12
MANGO SMOOTHIE	12
HOT CHOCOLATE	13
BERRY CHIA PUDDING	13
APPLE CHIA PUDDING	14
CHOCOLATE-TASTED CHIA PUDDING	14
FRUITY YOGURT PARFAIT	15
PEACH OATMEAL	16
PROTEIN OATMEAL	17
GREEN TEA OATMEAL	17
CREAMY OATMEAL	18
QUINOA PORRIDGE	18
CHOCOLATY QUINOA PORRIDGE	19
MILLET PORRIDGE	20
NUTTY GRANOLA	21
OAT GRANOLA	22
OAT & NUTS GRANOLA	23
FRUITY SEEDS BARS	24
CITRUS BARS	25
DRIED FRUIT BARS	26
CHOCOLATY OAT BARS	27
PROTEIN BARS	28
3-INGREDIENTS COOKIES	29
CHOCOLATY OAT COOKIES	30
BLUEBERRIES COOKIES	31
COFFEE COOKIES	32

Fruit Muffins	33
Oat Muffins	34
Jalapeño Muffins	35
Hash Brown Muffins	36
Muffin Sandwich	37
Apple Bread	38
Cranberry Bread	39
Chocolate Bread	40
Cheesy Onion Bread	41
Veggie Bread	42
Blueberry Pancakes	43
Butter Pancakes	44
Savory Pancakes	45
Oat Waffles	46
Pumpkin Waffles	47
Chocolate Waffles	48
Veggies & Egg Bowl	49
Kale & Egg Bowl	50
Sausage & Beans Bowl	51
Broccoli Omelet	52
Asparagus Frittata	53
Sausage Casserole	54
Lunch Recipes	55
Watermelon Salad	56
Apple Salad	57
Pomegranate & Apple Salad	58
Berries Salad	59
Mixed Fruit Salad	60
Tropical Fruit Salad	61

Rainbow Veggie Salad	62
Zucchini Noodles Salad	63
Zucchini & Cucumber Salad	64
Tofu & Veggie Salad	65
Quinoa & Kale Salad	66
Barley & Cherries Salad	67
Pasta Salad	68
Shrimp & Orange Salad	69
Tuna & Egg Salad	70
Tuna & Veggie Salad	71
Crab & Rice Salad	72
Creamy Apple Soup	73
Apple & Spinach Soup	73
Peach Soup	74
Cherry Soup	74
Strawberry & Rhubarb Soup	75
Mixed Fruit Soup	75
Quinoa & Berry Soup	76
Beet Soup	76
Zucchini Soup	77
Split Pea & Kale Soup	77
Beans & Artichoke Soup	78
Asparagus Soup	79
Broccoli Soup	80
Cauliflower Soup	81
Sweet Potato Soup	82
Carrot Soup	83
Peas Soup	84
Spinach Soup	85

Tomato Soup	86
Broccoli & Watercress Soup	87
Greens Soup	88
Mushroom Soup	89
Pumpkin Soup	90
Bell Pepper Soup	91
Green Veggie Soup	92
Sweet & Spicy Meatballs	93
Meatballs with Apple Sauce	94
Meatballs with Yogurt Dip	95
Chicken & Oat Burgers	96
Turkey & Apple Burgers	97
Beef & Veggie Burgers	98
Salmon Burgers	99
Beans & Veggie Burgers	100
Chicken Pitas	101
Chicken & Beans Bowl	102
Sausage & Beans Bowl	103
Pork & Beans Bowl	104
Beans & Rice Burritos	105
Glazed Shrimp	106
Shrimp with Zucchini	107
Prawns with Veggies	108
Scallops with Asparagus	109
Curried Potatoes	110
Curried Okra	111
Cauliflower with Peas	112
Veggies Stir-Fry	113
Veggies with Apple	114

ROASTED VEGGIES	115
ROASTED CHICKPEAS & VEGGIES	116
POTATO WITH CHICKPEAS	117
MUSHROOM WITH CORN	118
TOFU WITH BRUSSELS SPROUT	119
TOFU WITH VEGGIES	120
TEMPEH IN TOMATO SAUCE	121
SPICY QUINOA	123
QUINOA WITH EDAMAME	124
LENTILS WITH TOMATOES	125
PUMPKIN MACARONI	126
DINNER RECIPES	127
CHEESY CHICKEN SALAD	128
CHICKEN & CRANBERRY SALAD	129
CHICKEN & FRUIT SALAD	130
CHICKEN & FARO SALAD	131
CHICKEN & CHICKPEAS SALAD	133
TURKEY & PASTA SALAD	134
GROUND TURKEY SALAD	135
TURKEY & CHICKPEAS SALAD	136
STEAK SALAD	137
GROUND BEEF SALAD	138
PORK & GRAPES SALAD	139
PORK & VEGGIE SALAD	140
MEAT & VEGGIE SALAD	141
SHRIMP & VEGGIE SALAD	142
GRAINS & MANGO SALAD	144
GRAINS & SWEET POTATO SALAD	146
CHICKPEAS & VEGGIE SALAD	147

Chickpeas & Lentil Salad	148
Beans & Mango Salad	149
Beans & Corn Salad	150
Couscous & Beans Salad	151
Quinoa & Chickpeas Salad	152
Quinoa & Veggies Salad	153
Wheat Berries Salad	154
Soba Noodles Salad	156
Rice & Mango Salad	157
Rice & Tofu Salad	158
Curried Chicken Soup	159
Creamy Chicken Soup	160
Chicken & Potato Soup	161
Chicken & Sweet Potato Soup	162
Chicken & Veggie Soup	163
Chicken & Noodles Soup	164
Chicken & Quinoa Soup	165
Turkey & Spinach Soup	166
Beef & Mushroom Soup	167
Beef & Barley Soup	168
Pork & Sweet Potato Soup	169
Sausage & Beans Soup	170
Salmon & Cabbage Soup	171
Shrimp & Bell Pepper Soup	172
Mussels & Corn Soup	173
Barley & Beans Soup	174
Beans & Greens Soup	175
Beans & Broccoli Soup	176
Two-Beans Soup	177

LENTIL & VEGGIE SOUP	178
QUINOA & CARROT SOUP	179
LENTIL & QUINOA SOUP	180
ROOT VEGGIES SOUP	181
CHICKEN & CHICKPEAS STEW	182
BEEF & PUMPKIN STEW	183
BEEF & SQUASH STEW	184
LAMB STEW	185
HADDOCK STEW	186
SEAFOOD STEW	187
CHICKPEAS & SQUASH STEW	188
MIXED VEGGIE STEW	189
VEGGIES & RICE STEW	190
BEE CURRY	191
SALMON CURRY	192
MUSHROOM & CORN CURRY	193
LENTIL & APPLE CURRY	194
CASHEW CHICKEN	195
CHICKEN & VEGGIES	197
CHICKEN WITH CAULIFLOWER RICE	198
STUFFED CHICKEN CUTLETS	199
MINI CHICKEN PIES	200
BEEF IN MILKY SAUCE	201
CHICKEN SAUSAGE WITH VEGGIES	202
PORK WITH PINEAPPLE	203
LAMB WITH COUSCOUS	204
VEGGIES COMBO	205
MINI VEGGIES PIES	206
MIXED GRAINS COMBO	208

Breakfast Recipes

Green Pina Colada Smoothie

2 cups fresh pineapple chunks

2 cups fresh baby spinach

2 teaspoons raw honey

1 banana, peeled and sliced

1 cup unsweetened coconut mil

> In 2 meal prep containers, divide pineapple, banana and spinach. Cover and store in freezer for about 2-3 days.

> just before serving, remove containers from freezer and transfer the pineapple mixture in a high-speed blender. Add coconut milk and honey and pulse until smooth. Transfer into 2 serving glasses and serve immediately.

Servings **2**   Per Serving: Calories **439**   Protein **29.1g**   Carbohydrates **48.8g**   Fat **29.1g**

Chocolate Smoothie

2 cups frozen blueberries

2 tablespoons cacao powder

2 scoops vanilla protein powder

1 cup unsweetened almond milk

3 cups frozen spinach

2 tablespoons hemp seeds, hulled

2 teaspoons spirulina

> In 2 meal prep containers, divide all ingredients except almond milk. Cover and store in freezer for about 2-3 days.

> just before serving, remove containers from freezer and transfer the pineapple mixture in a high-speed blender. Add almond milk and pulse until smooth. Transfer into 2 serving glasses and serve immediately.

Servings **2**   Per Serving: Calories **490**   Protein **79g**   Carbohydrates **30.5g**   Fat **10.5g**

Protein Smoothie

2/3 cup rolled oats

2 medium bananas, peeled and sliced

3 oranges, peeled, seeded and sectioned

2½ cups unsweetened almond milk

1/8 teaspoon ground cinnamon

> In a high-speed blender, add all ingredients and pulse until smooth. Transfer the smoothie into 2 mason jars, leaving some place at the top. Cover tightly with a lid and freeze.

> Remove the jars from freezer and keep side at room temperature to thaw before serving.

Servings **4**   Per Serving: Calories **194**   Protein **4.g**   Carbohydrates **40.2g**   Fat **3.4g**

Mango Smoothie

1½ cups fresh mango, peeled, pitted and chopped

1 large banana, peeled and sliced

½ cup coconut yogurt

1 cup coconut water

> In a high-speed blender, add all ingredients and pulse until smooth. Transfer the smoothie into 2 mason jars, leaving some place at the top. Cover tightly with a lid and freeze.

> Remove the jars from freezer and keep side at room temperature to thaw before serving.

Servings **2**   Per Serving: Calories **161**   Protein **2.9g**   Carbohydrates **39.1g**   Fat **0.9g**

Hot Chocolate

1 cup granulated sugar

1 cup unsweetened cocoa powder

¼ teaspoon salt

12 cups boiling water

1 cup powdered milk

½ cup mini chocolate chips

½ cup mini marshmallows

> In a wide mouth mason jar layer the sugar, powdered milk, cocoa powder, chocolate chips, salt and marshmallows. Cover tightly with a lid and preserve in refrigerator.

> In Just before serving, transfer the chocolate mixture into a bowl and stir to combine. Divide chocolate mixture in 12 mugs. Pour hot water and stir to combine. Serve hot.

Servings **12**   Per Serving: *Calories* **166**   *Protein* **6.1g**   *Carbohydrates* **32.8g**   *Fat* **3.1g**

Berry Chia Pudding

2 tablespoons blueberries

2 tablespoons raspberries

1 tablespoon honey

2 tablespoons blackberries

2 tablespoons chia seeds

1 cup skim milk

> In a bowl, add all ingredients and stir to combine.

> Transfer mixture into 2 mason jars. Cover tightly and shake well.

> Refrigerate overnight.

Servings **2**   Per Serving: *Calories* **74**   *Protein* **1.8g**   *Carbohydrates* **14,7g**   *Fat* **2.6g**

Apple Chia Pudding

1 cup unsweetened almond milk

4 tablespoons chia seeds

1 teaspoon ground cinnamon, divided

¼ teaspoon vanilla extract

2 apples, cored and chopped finely

1 teaspoon raw honey

3 teaspoons water

3 tablespoons golden raisins

> In a bowl, mix together almond milk, chia seeds, ½ teaspoon of cinnamon and vanilla extract. Refrigerate for about 1 hour.

> In a microwave safe bowl, mix together apple, honey, water and remaining cinnamon and microwave on High for about 1-2 minutes, stirring once. Remove from microwave and stir in raisins. Add half of apple mixture in chia seeds mixture and stir to combine.

> Transfer mixture into 2 mason jars. Cover tightly and shake well.

> Refrigerate overnight.

Servings **2** Per Serving: Calories **250** Protein **4.6g** Carbohydrates **52.4g** Fat **7.2g**

Chocolate-Tasted Chia Pudding

6-8 dates, pitted and chopped

1½ cups unsweetened almond milk

1/3 cup chia seeds

¼ cup unsweetened cocoa powder

½ teaspoon ground cinnamon

Salt, to taste

½ teaspoon vanilla extract

> In a food processor, add all ingredients and pulse until smooth.

> Transfer mixture into 2 mason jars. Cover tightly and shake well. Refrigerate overnight.

Servings **4** Per Serving: Calories **103** Protein **3.8g** Carbohydrates **17.3g** Fat **5.4g**

Fruity Yogurt Parfait

12-ounce plain Greek yogurt

¼ cup almond milk

1/3 cup old-fashioned oats

1 teaspoon chia seeds

1 cup frozen strawberries

> In a bowl, add yogurt, almond milk, oats and chia seeds and stir until well combined. In 2 wide mouth mason jars, divide half of yogurt mixture and top with half strawberries. Repeat the layers once.

> Refrigerate up to 2-3 days.

Servings **2**   Per Serving**:**   *Calories* **269**   *Protein* **19.8g**   *Carbohydrates* **24.4g**   *Fat* **10.8g**

Peach Oatmeal

- 1 cup rolled oats
- 2 tablespoons ground flax seeds
- ½ teaspoon baking powder
- 1 teaspoon ground cinnamon
- ¼ teaspoon ground nutmeg
- Pinch of salt
- 1 cup almond milk
- 2 tablespoons pure maple syrup
- 1½ teaspoons vanilla extract
- 1 peach, pitted and chopped
- 1/3 cup walnuts, chopped

> Preheat your oven to 350 degrees F.

> In a large bowl, add oats, ground flax seeds, baking powder, spices and salt and mix well. Add almond milk, maple syrup and vanilla extract and mix until well combined. Fold in peach and walnuts. Transfer the mixture into 2 mason jars evenly, leaving some space from top. With your hands, gently press the oatmeal.

> Arrange the mason jars onto a large cookie sheet. Bake for 23 minutes or until top becomes golden brown.

> Remove from heat and keep aside to cool. Cover tightly with a lid and refrigerate to preserve.

Servings **2** Per Serving: Calories **693** Protein **15.2g** Carbohydrates **60.9g** Fat **46.1g**

Protein Oatmeal

3 cups quick cooking oatmeal

2 scoops vanilla protein powder

4 cups unsweetened almond milk

½ cup plain Greek yogurt

2 tablespoons chia seeds

Pinch of salt

1 teaspoon vanilla extract

> In a large bowl, add all ingredients except yogurt and mix until well combined. Refrigerate, covered overnight.

> In the morning, remove from refrigerator. Add yogurt and stir to combine before serving.

Servings **6** Per Serving: Calories **287** Protein **20g** Carbohydrates **33.6g** Fat **8.6g**

Green Tea Oatmeal

1 cup rolled oats

2 tablespoons chia seeds

1 cup light coconut milk

Pinch of salt

2 bananas, peeled and mashed

2 teaspoons matcha green tea

½ cup soy milk

2 tablespoons almonds, chopped

> In a large bowl, add all ingredients except almonds and mix until well combined. Refrigerate, covered overnight.

> In the morning, remove from refrigerator. Top with almonds and serve.

Servings **2** Per Serving: Calories **683** Protein **14.2g** Carbohydrates **82.4g** Fat **38.2g**

Creamy Oatmeal

1 cup rolled oats ½ cup fresh strawberries, hulled and chopped

1 teaspoon fresh lemon zest, grated finely 2 tablespoons chia seeds

1½ cups full-fat coconut milk ¾ cup plain Greek yogurt

1/3 cup cream cheese, softened 2 teaspoons fresh lemon juice

½ teaspoon vanilla extract 2 tablespoons honey

> In a medium bowl, add all ingredients and mix until well combined. Refrigerate, covered overnight.

> Serve in the morning.

Servings **2** Per Serving: Calories **832** Protein **17.6g** Carbohydrates **50.6g** Fat **67g**

Quinoa Porridge

2 cups unsweetened almond milk 1 cup quinoa

½ teaspoon ground cinnamon ¼ teaspoon ground cardamom

2 tablespoons maple syrup 4 cups mixed berries

4 tablespoons almonds, sliced

> In a medium pan, add almond milk, quinoa, cinnamon and cardamom and bring to a boil. Reduce heat and simmer for about 15 minutes.

> Remove from heat and keep aside to cool. After cooling, stir in maple syrup. Divide quinoa mixture into 4 containers, followed by berries and almonds. Refrigerate for 1-2 days.

> Remove from refrigerator and re-heat in microwave before serving.

Servings **4** Per Serving: Calories **318** Protein **8.8g** Carbohydrates **53.6g** Fat **7.8g**

Chocolaty Quinoa Porridge

1 cup water

½ cup quinoa

2/3 cup chocolate soy milk

1 tablespoon cocoa powder

1 tablespoon maple syrup

1 banana, peeled and mashed

> In a pan, add water and quinoa over medium heat and cook for about five minutes. Add soy milk and stir to combine. Reduce the heat to medium-low and simmer for about 5-7 minutes or until most of liquid is absorbed.

> Remove from heat and stir in cocoa powder, maple syrup and banana slices. Keep aside to cool. After cooling, stir in maple syrup. Divide quinoa mixture into 2 containers, followed by berries and almonds. Refrigerate for 1-2 days.

> Remove from refrigerator and re-heat in microwave before serving.

Servings **2**   Per Serving: *Calories* **285**   *Protein* **16.5g**   *Carbohydrates* **54.1g**   *Fat* **4.6g**

Millet Porridge

1 cup millet, rinsed and drained

3 cups water

6-8 drops liquid stevia

4 tablespoons fresh blueberries

Pinch of salt

2 tablespoons almonds, chopped finely

1 cup unsweetened almond milk

> Heat a non-stick pan over medium-low heat and toast millet for about 2-3 minutes, stirring continuously. Add salt and water and bring to a boil over medium heat. Cook for about 15 minutes. Stir in almonds, stevia and almond milk and cook for 4-5 minutes more.

> Remove from heat and keep aside to cool. After cooling, stir in maple syrup. Divide millet mixture into 4 containers, followed by berries and almonds. Refrigerate for 1-2 days.

> Remove from refrigerator and re-heat in microwave before serving. Top with blueberries and serve.

Servings | **4**   Per Serving: *Calories* | **221**   *Protein* | **6.5g**   *Carbohydrates* | **38.9g**   *Fat* | **4.5g**

Nutty Granola

- 1 cup almonds
- 1 cup walnuts
- ¼ cup unsweetened cocoa powder
- ¼ cup walnut oil
- 2-ounce chocolate, chopped
- 1 cup hazelnuts
- 1 cup flax seeds meal
- Salt, to taste
- ¼ cup almond butter, melted
- ½ cup swerve (sugar substitute)

> Preheat the oven to 300 degrees F. Line a large rimmed baking sheet with parchment paper.

> In a food processor, add almonds, hazelnuts and walnuts and pulse until a coarse crumb like mixture forms. Transfer the nut mixture into a large bowl. Add flax seeds meal, cocoa powder and salt and mix well.

> In a pan, add walnut oil, butter and chocolate over low heat. Cook for about 2-3 minutes or until smooth, stirring continuously. Stir in swerve and immediately, remove from heat. Add the butter mixture over nut mixture and toss to coat well. Place the mixture onto prepared baking sheet evenly.

> Bake for about 15 minutes, stirring after every 5 minutes.

> Turn off the oven but keep the baking sheet in oven for about 20 minutes, stirring occasionally.

> Remove from oven and keep aside to cool completely.

> Transfer granola in an airtight container and store in a cool, dry place for up to 2 weeks.

Servings **10** Per Serving**:** *Calories* **479** *Protein* **9.2g** *Carbohydrates* **24.4g** *Fat* **44.2g**

Oat Granola

2 cups old fashion oats

¼ cup sunflower seeds

2-3 tablespoons maple syrup

½ teaspoon vanilla extract

½ cup raw walnuts, chopped

½ cup unsweetened dried cherries

2 tablespoons virgin coconut oil

Pinch of fine sea salt

> Preheat the oven to 300 degrees F.

> In a large bowl, add all ingredients and mix well. Place the mixture onto a baking sheet in a thin layer.

> Remove from oven and keep aside to cool completely.

> Transfer granola in an airtight container and store in a cool, dry place for up to 2 weeks.

Servings | **6**   Per Serving: *Calories* | **266**   *Protein* | **6.2g**   *Carbohydrates* | **30.7g**   *Fat* | **14.2g**

Oat & Nuts Granola

8 cups rolled oats

1½ cups oat bran

1½ cups wheat germ

1 cup sunflower seeds

1 cup walnuts, chopped finely

1 cup pecans, chopped finely

1 cup almonds, chopped finely

1 cup vegetable oil

½ cup brown sugar

¾ cup honey

¼ cup maple syrup

1 tablespoon vanilla extract

1 tablespoon ground cinnamon

1½ teaspoons salt

2 cups raisins

> Preheat the oven to 325 degrees F. Line 2 large baking sheets with parchment papers.

> In a large bowl, mix together oats, oat bran, wheat germ, sunflower seeds and nuts.

> In a pan, mix together oil, brown sugar, honey, maple syrup, vanilla extract, cinnamon and salt over medium heat and bring to a boil. Immediately, remove from heat. Pour oil mixture over oat mixture and stir to combine. Spread oat mixture onto prepared baking sheets evenly.

> Bake for about 20 minutes, stirring once in the middle way. Remove from oven and keep aside to cool. After, cooling, stir in raisins.

> Transfer granola in an airtight container and store in a cool, dry place for up to 2 weeks.

Servings **30**   Per Serving: Calories **331**   Protein **7.8g**   Carbohydrates **40.7g**   Fat **17/4g**

Fruity Seeds Bars

1 (12-ounce) package whole cranberries

1 cup white sugar

¾ cup water

1 (18¼-ounce) package yellow cake mix

2 eggs

¾ cup melted butter

1 cup rolled oats

¾ cup light brown sugar

1 teaspoon ground cinnamon

1 teaspoon ground ginger

Pinch of ground cloves

Pinch of ground cardamom

> In a pan, add cranberries, sugar and water over medium heat and cook for about 15 minutes, stirring occasionally. Remove from heat and keep aside to cool completely.

> Preheat the oven to 350 degrees F. Lightly, grease a 13x9-inch baking dish.

> In a large bowl, add cake mix, eggs and butter and mix until well combined. Add oats, brown sugar and spices and stir to combine. Reserve about 1½ cups of the mixture in another bowl and keep aside.

> Place the remaining mixture into prepared baking dish and with the palm of your hands slightly, press downwards. Spread cranberry sauce over oat mixture evenly. Sprinkle with reserved oat mixture evenly.

> Bake for about 35-40 minutes or until top becomes golden brown.

> Remove from oven and keep onto a wire rack to cool. With a sharp knife, cut into desired sized bars.

> **Store** these bars in an airtight container, by placing parchment papers between the bars to avoid the sticking. These bars can be stored in the refrigerator for up to 2 weeks.

Servings **24**   Per Serving**:**   Calories **219**   Protein **1.9g**   Carbohydrates **33.4g**   Fat **8.8g**

Citrus Bars

2¼ cups all-purpose flour, divided

1 cup butter, softened

¼ cup fresh lemon juice

2 cups white sugar, divided

4 eggs

> Preheat the oven to 350 degrees F.

> In a bowl add 2 cups of flour, ½ cup of sugar and butter and mix until well combined. Transfer the mixture into a 13x9-inch ungreased baking dish evenly and with the back of a spatula, press in the bottom.

> Bake for about 15-20 minutes.

> Remove from oven and keep onto a wire rack to cool.

> Meanwhile in another bowl, mix together remaining flour and remaining sugar. Add eggs and lemon juice and beat until well combined. Place the egg mixture over baked crust evenly and with the back of a spatula, smooth the top surface.

> Bake for about 20 minutes or until top becomes golden brown.

> Remove from oven and keep onto a wire rack to cool. With a sharp knife, cut into desired sized bars.

> Store these bars in an airtight container, by placing parchment papers between the bars to avoid the sticking. These bars can be stored in the refrigerator for up to 2 weeks.

Servings 36   Per Serving: *Calories* 123   *Protein* 1.5g   *Carbohydrates* 17.2g   *Fat* 5.7g

Dried Fruit Bars

1 cup dried figs, quartered and divided

1 cup dried apricots, chopped and divided

1/3 cup light brown sugar

1/8 teaspoon baking soda

¼ teaspoon salt

1 large egg

½ cup dried cranberries, divided

1/3 cup whole-grain flour

1/8 teaspoon baking powder

½ teaspoon ground cinnamon

1½ cups walnuts, toasted and chopped

1 teaspoon vanilla extract

> Preheat the oven to 325 degrees F. Line an 8x8-inch baking dish with parchment paper.

> In a food processor, add half of each dry fruit, flour, brown sugar, baking soda, baking powder, cinnamon and salt and pulse until well combined. Transfer the mixture into a large bowl. Add remaining dry fruit and walnuts and mix well.

> In a small bowl, add egg and vanilla extract and beat well. Add egg mixture into walnut mixture and mix until well combined. Place mixture into prepared baking dish evenly and with the back of a spatula, smooth the top surface.

> Bake for about 35-40 minutes or until top becomes golden brown.

> Remove from oven and keep on wire rack to cool. With a sharp knife, cut into desired sized bars.

> Store these bars in an airtight container, by placing parchment papers between the bars to avoid the sticking. These bars can be stored in the refrigerator for up to 2 weeks.

Servings **12**   Per Serving: Calories **180**   Protein **5.5g**   Carbohydrates **20.5g**   Fat **9.9g**

Chocolaty Oat Bars

1½ cups rolled oats

½ cup cashews, chopped roughly

1/3 cup pumpkin seeds

¼ cup sunflower seeds

2 tablespoons chia seeds

½ cup agave nectar

½ cup almonds, chopped roughly

½ cup mini chocolate chips

¼ cup sesame seeds

¼ cup flaxseed meal

1 teaspoon ground cinnamon

1 cup almond butter, softened

> Line an 8x8-inch baking dish with a large lightly greased parchment paper.

> In a large bowl, add oats, nuts, chocolate chips, seeds and cinnamon and mix well. Add agave nectar and stir to combine. Add almond butter and mix until well combined.

> Place oat mixture into prepared baking dish evenly and with the back of a spatula, smooth the top surface, by pressing in the bottom. Refrigerate for about 6-8 hours or until set completely.

Remove from refrigerator and with a sharp knife, cut into desired sized bars.

> Store these bars in an airtight container, by placing parchment papers between the bars to avoid the sticking. These bars can be stored in the refrigerator for up to 2 weeks.

Servings **12**   Per Serving**:**   *Calories* **241**   *Protein* **6.2g**   *Carbohydrates* **27.2g**   *Fat* **13g**

Protein Bars

1 cup rice Krispies

¼ cup oat flour

3 tablespoons almond butter

1/8 teaspoon salt

1 scoop vanilla protein powder

5 tablespoons agave nectar

1 teaspoon vanilla extract

½ cup dried strawberries, chopped finely

> Line a bread loaf pan with parchment paper.

> In a large bowl, mix together rice Krispies, protein powder and oat flour. In another small bowl, add remaining ingredients except strawberries and mix until well combined. Add almond butter mixture into flour mixture and mix until well combined. Fold in strawberries.

> Place the mixture into prepared loaf pan evenly and with the back of a spatula, smooth the top surface, by pressing in the bottom. Refrigerate for about 2 hours or until set completely.

> Remove from refrigerator and with a sharp knife, cut into desired sized bars.

> **Store** these bars in an airtight container, by placing parchment papers between the bars to avoid the sticking. These bars **can be stored in the refrigerator for up to 2 weeks.**

Servings **8**   Per Serving: Calories **135**   Protein **5.7g**   Carbohydrates **19.3g**   Fat **4.3g**

3-Ingredients Cookies

¾ cup coconut, shredded

1 banana, peeled and sliced

Pinch of ground cinnamon

> Preheat the oven to 350 degrees F. Grease a cookie sheet.

> In a food processor, add all ingredients and pulse until smooth. Spoon the mixture onto prepared cookie sheet. Gently, press the cookies.

> Bake for about 25 minutes or until golden brown.

> Remove from oven and keep onto a wire rack to cool for about 5 minutes. Carefully, invert cookies onto wire rack to cool completely.

> Store these cookies in an airtight container, by placing parchment papers between the cookies to avoid the sticking. These cookies can be stored in the refrigerator for up to 2 weeks.

Servings **5** Per Serving**:** *Calories* **64** *Protein* **0.7g** *Carbohydrates* **7.3g** *Fat* **4.1g**

Chocolaty Oat Cookies

1 tablespoon ground flaxseed meal

2½ tablespoons warm water

2 cups oat flour

1 cup whole rolled oats

1 teaspoon baking soda

1 teaspoon ground cinnamon

¼ teaspoon ground nutmeg

¼ teaspoon s salt

¾ cup canned pumpkin puree

¾ cup cane sugar

½ cup warm coconut oil. Melted

1 teaspoon vanilla extract

1 cup chocolate chips

> Preheat the oven to 350 degrees F. Line a large cookie sheet with parchment paper.

> In a small bowl, mix together flaxseeds and water and keep aside until thicken.

> In a large bowl, mix together oat flour, oats, baking soda, spices and salt. In another bowl, add pumpkin, sugar, coconut oil and vanilla extract and beat until well combined. Add flaxseed mixture and stir to combine. Add pumpkin mixture into flour mixture and mix until well combined. Fold in chocolate chips. With a large cookie scoop, place mixture onto prepared cookie sheet.

> Bake for about 16-19 minutes or until the tops become browned.

> Remove from oven and keep onto a wire rack to cool for about 5 minutes. Carefully, invert cookies onto wire rack to cool completely.

> Store these cookies in an airtight container, by placing parchment papers between the cookies to avoid the sticking. These cookies can be stored in the refrigerator for up to 2 weeks.

Servings **12**   Per Serving: Calories **296**   Protein **4.3g**   Carbohydrates **37.6g**   Fat **14.9g**

Blueberries Cookies

1½ cups rolled oats

¾ cup pecans, chopped roughly

1 tablespoon golden flax meal

3 ripe bananas, peeled and mashed

1 tablespoon honey

1 cup unsweetened coconut flakes

½ cup dried blueberries

½ teaspoon salt

¼ cup coconut oil, melted

1 teaspoon vanilla extract

> Preheat the oven to 350 degrees F. Grease age cookie sheet.

> In a large bowl, mix together oats, coconut, pecans, blueberries, flax meal and salt. Add remaining ingredients and mix until well combined.

> Place dough onto a lightly floured surface and with a 2½-inch round cookie cutter, cut cookies. Arrange cookies onto prepared cookie sheet in a single layer.

> Bake for about 25 minutes or until golden.

> Remove from oven and keep onto a wire rack to cool for about 5 minutes. Carefully, invert cookies onto wire rack to cool completely.

> Store these cookies in an airtight container, by placing parchment papers between the cookies to avoid the sticking. These cookies can be stored in the refrigerator for up to 2 weeks.

Servings **15**   Per Serving: *Calories* **156**   *Protein* **2.4g**   *Carbohydrates* **14.9g**   *Fat* **10.6g**

Coffee Cookies

1/3 cup shortening

½ cup white sugar

1½ teaspoons vanilla extract

2 cups all-purpose flour

¼ teaspoon baking soda

2 tablespoon instant coffee powder

½ cup packed brown sugar

1 egg

1 tablespoon milk

½ teaspoon salt

¼ teaspoon baking powder

> Preheat the oven to 400 degrees F. Line cookie sheets with the parchment papers.

> In a bowl, add the shortening, brown sugar, white sugar, egg, vanilla and milk and beat until fluffy. In another bowl, mix together flour, salt, baking soda, baking powder and instant coffee. Add the flour mixture into the sugar mixture and mix until well combined. Make about 1-inch balls from the mixture. Place balls on the prepared baking sheets in a single layer about 2-inch apart. With the sugar dipped fork, flatten the cookies to 1/8-inch thickness.

> Bake for about 8-10 minutes or until top becomes golden brown.

> Remove from oven and keep onto a wire rack to cool for about 5 minutes. Carefully, invert cookies onto wire rack to cool completely.

> Store these cookies in an airtight container, by placing parchment papers between the cookies to avoid the sticking. These cookies can be stored in the refrigerator for up to 2 weeks.

Servings | **12**   Per Serving**:** *Calories* | **192**   *Protein* | **2.7g**   *Carbohydrates* | **30.5g**   *Fat* | **6.3g**

Fruit Muffins

2 cups all-purpose flour
1 teaspoon baking soda
½ teaspoon ground nutmeg
½ teaspoon ground cinnamon
Pinch of ground ginger
Pinch of ground cloves
¼ teaspoon sea salt
1¼ cups white sugar
2/3 cup shortening
3 eggs
¼ cup buttermilk
1 teaspoon vanilla extract
2 apples, peeled, cored and shredded
1 cup banana, peeled and mashed

> Preheat the oven to 375 degrees F. Line 24 cups of mini muffin tins with paper liners.

> In a large bowl, mix together flour, baking soda, spices and salt. In another bowl, add sugar and shortening and beat until fluffy and light. Add eggs, one at a time and beat until well combined. Add buttermilk and vanilla extract and beat until well combined. Add flour mixture and mix until just combined. Fold in apples and banana. Transfer the mixture in prepared muffin cups evenly.

> Bake for about 20-25 minutes or until a tooth pick inserted in the center comes out clean.

> Remove the muffin tins from oven and keep on wire rack to cool for about 10 minutes. Carefully turn on a wire rack to cool completely.

> Line 1-2 airtight container with paper towels. Arrange muffins over paper towel in a single layer. Cover muffins with another paper towel. Refrigerate for about 2-3 days. Reheat in the microwave on High for about 2 minutes before serving.

Servings **12**   Per Serving**:**   Calories **305**   Protein **4g**   Carbohydrates **45.2g**   Fat **12.9g**

Oat Muffins

¼ cup unsalted butter

1 tablespoon instant coffee powder

1 teaspoon salt

2/3 cup milk

1 cup pecans, chopped

2½ cups rolled oats

2 teaspoons baking powder

3 eggs

2/3 cup maple syrup

¾ cup dried cherries, chopped roughly

> Preheat the oven to 400 degrees F. Line 12 cups of a muffin tin with greased paper liners.

> In a small skillet, add butter over medium heat and melt until browned. Remove from heat and keep aside to cool.

> Meanwhile, in a bowl, mix together oats, coffee powder, baking powder and salt. In another bowl, add eggs, milk and maple syrup and beat until well combined. Add cooled butter and beat until well combined. Add egg mixture into oat mixture and mix until well combined. Keep aside for about 10 minutes, stirring occasionally. Now, fold in pecans and cherries. Transfer the mixture into prepared muffin cups evenly and with a back of spoon, smooth the top surface.

> Bake for about 35-50 minutes or until a toothpick inserted in the center comes out clean.

> Remove the muffin tins from oven and keep on wire rack to cool for about 10 minutes. Carefully turn on a wire rack to cool completely.

> Line 1-2 airtight container with paper towels. Arrange muffins over paper towel in a single layer. Cover muffins with another paper towel. Refrigerate for about 2-3 days. Reheat in the microwave on High for about 2 minutes before serving.

Servings **12**   Per Serving: Calories **244**   Protein **5,2g**   Carbohydrates **26.5g**   Fat **13.8g**

Jalapeño Muffins

1½ cups all-purpose flour

1 tablespoon granulated sugar

1 tablespoon baking powder

½ teaspoon salt

1 cup whole milk

¼ cup unsalted butter, melted

1 egg

3 cups sharp cheddar cheese, grated

3 tablespoons pickled jalapeño, chopped

> Preheat the oven to 375 degrees F. Line a 12-cups muffin pan with silicone liners.

> In a large bowl, mix together flour, sugar, baking powder and salt. In another bowl, add milk, butter and egg and beat until well combined. Add egg mixture into flour mixture and mix until just combined. Fold in cheese and jalapeño. Transfer the mixture in prepared muffin cups evenly.

> Bake for about 22-25 minutes or until top becomes golden brown.

> Remove the muffin tins from oven and keep on wire rack to cool for about 10 minutes. Carefully turn on a wire rack to cool completely.

> Line 1-2 airtight container with paper towels. Arrange muffins over paper towel in a single layer. Cover muffins with another paper towel. Refrigerate for about 2-3 days. Reheat in the microwave on High for about 2 minutes before serving.

Servings | **12**   Per Serving**:**   *Calories* | **227**   *Protein* | **9.8g**   *Carbohydrates* | **14.8g**   *Fat* | **14.4g**

Hash Brown Muffins

4 cups shredded hash browns, thawed
3 tablespoons olive oil
Salt and ground black pepper, to taste
2 tablespoons butter
1½ cups leeks, chopped
½ cup yellow onion, chopped
7 eggs, beaten
2 cups cheddar cheese, shredded
6-ounce canned corned beef, chopped
Salt and freshly ground black pepper, to taste

> Preheat the oven to 400 F. Line a 12-cups muffin pan with silicone liners.

> In a bowl, mix together hash browns, oil, salt and black pepper. Place hash brown mixture into each prepared muffin cup and press slightly in the bottom.

> Bake for about 30-40 minutes or until golden.

> meanwhile, in a skillet, melt butter over medium-high heat and cook leeks and onions for about 6-7 minutes. Remove from heat and keep aside to cool.

> In a bowl, eggs, cheese, salt and black pepper and beat until well combined.

> Remove muffin tin from oven and top each cup with corned beef, followed by cooked leek mixture and egg mixture evenly.

> Bake for about 18-20 minutes.

> Remove the muffin tins from oven and keep on wire rack to cool for about 10 minutes. Carefully turn on a wire rack to cool completely.

> Line 1-2 airtight container with paper towels. Arrange muffins over paper towel in a single layer. Cover muffins with another paper towel. Refrigerate for about 2-3 days. Reheat in the microwave on High for about 2 minutes before serving.

Servings **12**   Per Serving**:**   *Calories* **348**   *Protein* **12.1g**   *Carbohydrates* **24.9g**   *Fat* **22.6g**

Muffin Sandwich

6 large eggs

Salt and freshly ground black pepper, to taste

6 English muffins, slice in half

6 cheddar cheese slices

6 deli ham slices

> Preheat the oven to 350 degrees F. Grease 6 ramekins and arrange onto a baking sheet.

> Carefully, crack 1 egg in each ramekin. With a fork, pierce yolk of each egg and then, beat slightly. Sprinkle with salt and black pepper.

> Bake for about 12-15 minutes or until set.

> Remove from oven and keep aside to cool completely. After cooling, carefully remove eggs from ramekins.

> Arrange 6 muffin halves onto a smooth surface. Place 1 cheese slices over each muffin half, followed by ham slice and egg. Top with remaining muffin halves.

> With a plastic wrap, cover each muffin sandwich and freeze for up to 2 days. Reheat in the microwave on High for about 2 minutes before serving.

Servings **6**   Per Serving**:**   *Calories* **238**   *Protein* **15.3g**   *Carbohydrates* **26.6g**   *Fat* **7.7g**

Apple Bread

1 cup whole-wheat flour	½ cup quick oats
1 teaspoon baking soda	½ teaspoon baking powder
¼ teaspoon pumpkin spice	½ teaspoon ground cinnamon
Salt, to taste	¾ cup brown sugar
2 tablespoons butter, softened	1½ cups unsweetened applesauce
2 large egg whites	1 teaspoon vanilla extract
1 large apple, peeled, cored and chopped	1 cup almonds, chopped

> Preheat the oven to 325 degrees F. Grease 8 wide mouth mason jars with cooking spray.

> In a large bowl mix together flour, oats, baking soda, baking powder, pumpkin pie spice, cinnamon and salt. In another bowl, add brown sugar and butter and beat until well combined. Add applesauce, egg whites and vanilla extract and beat until fluffy and light. Slowly, add flour mixture in butter mixture, beating continuously until well combined. Gently, fold in apple and almonds. Place the mixture into prepared mason jars about ½ of full.

> Arrange the mason jars onto a large baking sheet. Bake for about 40-45 minutes or until a toothpick inserted in the center comes out clean.

> Remove from oven and keep onto wire racks to cool completely.

> Cover the mason jars with lid tightly. This bread can be stored in freezer for about 1 week.

Servings **8** Per Serving: Calories **167** Protein **3.6g** Carbohydrates **25.3g** Fat **8.9g**

Cranberry Bread

2 cups all-purpose flour

1½ teaspoons baking powder

¼ cup cold butter, chopped

¾ cup fresh orange juice

½ cup walnuts, chopped

¾ cup sugar

Salt, to taste

1 egg

1 cup fresh cranberries, chopped

1 tablespoon fresh orange zest, grated finely

> Preheat the oven to 350 degrees F. Grease an 8½x4½-inch bread loaf pan.

> In a large bowl, mix together flour, sugar, baking powder and salt. Add chopped butter and mix well. In another bowl, add egg, and beat well. Add orange juice and mix until well combined. Add egg mixture into flour mixture and mix until well combined. Gently, fold into cranberries, walnuts and orange zest. Transfer the mixture in prepared bread loaf pan evenly.

> Bake for about 60-75 minutes or until a toothpick inserted in the center comes out clean.

> Remove the bread pan from oven and keep onto a wire rack to cool for about 10 minutes. Carefully invert bread onto wire rack to cool completely. With a sharp knife, cut the bread loaf in desired sized slices.

> Store these bread slices in a large airtight container, by placing wax papers between the slices to avoid the sticking. This bread can be stored in the freezer for up to 3-4 days.

Servings **8**   Per Serving: *Calories* **313**   *Protein* **6g**   *Carbohydrates* **48.9g**   *Fat* **11.3g**

Chocolate Bread

1 ¾ cups all-purpose flour

½ cup unsweetened cocoa powder

½ teaspoon baking soda

½ teaspoon baking powder

Salt, to taste

1 cup sugar

½ cup butter, softened

2 eggs

1 cup buttermilk

1 teaspoon vanilla extract

1/3 cup walnuts, chopped

> Preheat the oven to 350 degrees F. Lightly, grease a 9x5-inch bead loaf pan.

> In a large bowl, mix together flour, cocoa powder, baking soda, baking powder and salt. In another bowl, add sugar and butter beat until creamy. Add eggs and beat well. Stir in buttermilk and vanilla extract. Add egg mixture into flour mixture and mix until just moistened. Gently, fold in walnuts. Transfer the bread mixture into prepared loaf pan evenly.

> Bake for about 55-65 minutes or until a toothpick inserted in the center comes out clean.

> Remove the bread pan from oven and keep onto a wire rack to cool for about 10 minutes. Carefully invert bread onto wire rack to cool completely. With a sharp knife, cut the bread loaf in desired sized slices.

> **Store** these bread slices in a large airtight container, by placing wax papers between the slices to avoid the sticking. This bread **can be stored in the freezer for up to 3-4 days.**

Servings **12**   Per Serving**:**   *Calories* **246**   *Protein* **5.1g**   *Carbohydrates* **34.1g**   *Fat* **11.3g**

Cheesy Onion Bread

1½ cups all-purpose flour

3 teaspoons baking powder

Salt and freshly ground black pepper, to taste

3 tablespoons cold butter, divided

1 cup sharp cheddar cheese, shredded and divided

½ cup onion, chopped finely

2 small garlic cloves, minced

½ cup milk

1 egg

> Preheat the oven to 400 degrees F. Grease an 8x8-inch square pan.

> In a large bowl, mix together flour, baking powder, salt and black pepper. With a pastry cutter, cut 2 tablespoons of butter until a crumbly mixture forms. Add ½ cup of cheese and stir to combine. Make a well in the center of flour mixture and keep aside.

> In a small frying pan, melt remaining butter over medium heat and sauté onion for about 3-4 minutes. Add garlic and sauté for about 20-30 seconds. Remove from heat and keep aside to cool slightly.

> In another bowl, add milk and eggs and beat well. Stir in onion mixture. Add onion mixture in the well of flour mixture and stir until just moistened. Transfer the bread mixture into prepared pan evenly. Top with the remaining cheese evenly.

> Bake for about 25 minutes or until a tooth pick inserted in the center comes out clean.

> Remove the bread pan from oven and keep onto a wire rack to cool for about 10 minutes. Carefully invert bread onto wire rack to cool completely. With a sharp knife, cut the bread loaf in desired sized slices.

> Store these bread slices in a large airtight container, by placing wax papers between the slices to avoid the sticking. This bread can be stored in the freezer for up to 3-4 days.

Servings **8**   Per Serving: *Calories* 202   *Protein* **2g**   *Carbohydrates* **20.7g**   *Fat* **10.1g**

Veggie Bread

2 cups unbleached all-purpose flour	½ cup cold unsalted butter, chopped
1 tablespoon baking powder	Salt, to taste
2 eggs	½ cup plain yogurt
6 scallions, chopped	1 cup zucchini, grated and squeezed
½ cup oil-packed black olives, drained, pitted and halved	
1 teaspoon fresh thyme, chopped	3½-ounce feta cheese, crumbled

> Preheat the oven to 350 degrees F. Line an 8x4-inch bread loaf pan with a lightly, greased parchment paper.

> In a food processor, add flour, butter, baking powder and salt and pulse until a sandy texture forms. Transfer the flour mixture into a large bowl.

> In another bowl, add eggs and yogurt and beat to combine. Add the egg mixture into flour mixture and mix until well combined. Add scallions, zucchini, olives and thyme and stir to combine. Fold in feta cheese. Transfer the bread mixture into prepared loaf pan evenly and with the back of a moistened spoon, smooth the top surface.

> Bake for about 75 minutes or until a tooth pick inserted in the center comes out clean.

> Remove the bread pan from oven and keep on wire rack to cool for about 10 minutes. Carefully invert bread onto wire rack to cool completely. With a sharp knife, cut the bread loaf in desired sized slices.

> **Store** these bread slices in a large airtight container, by placing wax papers between the slices to avoid the sticking. This bread can be stored in the freezer for up to 3-4 days.

Servings **8**   Per Serving**:**   Calories **293**   Protein **7.8g**   Carbohydrates **28.3g**   Fat **16.7g**

Blueberry Pancakes

1 cup flour

1 tablespoon baking powder

2 tablespoons unsalted butter, melted

2 tablespoons honey

2 tablespoons sugar

¾ cup milk

½ cup fresh blueberries

> In a bowl, mix together flour, sugar and baking powder. Add milk and butter and mux until a smooth mixture is formed.

> Divide the blueberries in 2 large mason jars evenly. Place the flour mixture over blueberries evenly. (Make sure to fill not more than ½ of the jar).

> Refrigerate overnight.

> In the morning, microwave on High for about 1½ minutes.

> Serve with topping of honey.

Servings **6**   Per Serving: *Calories* **171**   *Protein* **3.1g**   *Carbohydrates* **30.1g**   *Fat* **4.7g**

Butter Pancakes

1½ cups all-purpose flour, sifted

1 tablespoon white sugar

1¼ cups milk

3 tablespoons butter, melted

3½ teaspoons baking powder

1 teaspoon salt

1 egg

> In a large bowl, mix together the flour, baking powder, sugar and salt. Make a well in the center of flour mixture. In the well, place milk, egg and butter and mix until smooth.

> Heat a lightly greased griddle over medium-high heat. Add ¼ cup of mixture and cook until golden brown from both sides. Repeat with the remaining mixture.

> Remove from oven and keep aside to cool completely.

> **Store** these pancakes in a large airtight container, by placing wax papers between the pancakes to avoid the sticking. These pancakes **can be stored in the freezer for up to 2 weeks.**

Servings **8**   Per Serving**:**   *Calories* **158**   *Protein* **4.4g**   *Carbohydrates* **22.3g**   *Fat* **5.9g**

Savory Pancakes

½ cup tapioca flour

½ cup almond flour

½ teaspoon red chili powder

¼ teaspoon ground turmeric

Salt and freshly ground black pepper, to taste

1 cup coconut milk

½ of red onion, chopped

¼ teaspoon fresh ginger, grated finely

1 Serrano pepper, minced

½ cup fresh cilantro, chopped

> In a large bowl, combine together flours and spices and then add coconut milk and combine until well mixed. Put in the onion, ginger, Serrano pepper and cilantro.

> Gently grease a large non-stick skillet with oil and heat over medium heat. Add ¼ cup of mixture and tilt the pan to spread it evenly in the skillet. Cook for 4 minutes per side. Repeat with remaining mixture.

> Remove from your oven and keep to the side to cool fully.

> Store the pancakes in a large airtight container. Place wax papers between the pancakes to avoid sticking. These pancakes can be stored in the freezer for up to 2 weeks.

Servings | **6**   Per Serving: *Calories* | **218**   *Protein* | **3.1g**   *Carbohydrates* | **22.8g**   *Fat* | **14.3g**

Oat Waffles

2/3 cup oatmeal

½ teaspoon baking powder

¼ cup cottage cheese

1 teaspoon olive oil

1½ tablespoons powdered stevia

¼ cup egg substitute

½ cup water

½ teaspoon vanilla extract

> Preheat a waffle iron and grease it.

> In a food processor, add oatmeal, stevia and baking powder and blend until powdered fully. Put the mixture into a bowl.

> In the same food processor, add egg substitute, cottage cheese, water, oil and vanilla and blend until smooth. Transfer the mixture into the bowl with oatmeal mixture and mix until well combined.

> Add half of mixture into a waffle iron and cook for 4 minutes or according to manufacturer's instructions. Repeat with the remaining mixture.

> Store these waffles in a large airtight container. Place wax papers between the waffles to avoid sticking. These waffles can be stored in the freezer for up to 3 days.

Servings **2** Per Serving**:** *Calories* **170** *Protein* **11.2g** *Carbohydrates* **20.4g** *Fat* **4.7g**

Pumpkin Waffles

2½ cups all-purpose flour

4 teaspoons baking powder

1 teaspoon ground ginger

1 cup canned pumpkin

4 eggs, separated

¼ cup packed brown sugar

2 teaspoons ground cinnamon

½ teaspoon salt

2 cups milk

¼ cup butter, melted

> Preheat a waffle iron and grease it.

> In a large bowl, combine together flour, brown sugar, baking powder, spices and salt. In a different bowl, add pumpkin, milk and egg yolks and beat until fully mixed.

> In a smaller bowl, add egg whites and beat until soft peaks form. Add in flour mixture and butter into pumpkin mixture and mix until just combined. Using a rubber spatula, gently fold 1/3 of whipped egg whites into the pumpkin mixture. Put in remaining egg whites.

> Add desired amount of mixture into waffle iron and cook for 4 minutes or according to manufacturer's instructions. Repeat with remaining mixture.

> Store these waffles in a large airtight container. Place wax papers between the waffles to avoid the sticking. These waffles can be stored in the freezer for up to 3 days.

Servings **6**   Per Serving**:**   *Calories* **382**   *Protein* **12.3g**   *Carbohydrates* **56.6g**   *Fat* **12.9g**

Chocolate Waffles

1 cup all-purpose flour 1 cup whole wheat flour

¼ cup sugar ¼ cup cocoa powder

2 teaspoons baking powder 1 teaspoon baking soda

½ teaspoon salt 2 eggs (yolks and white separated)

1¼ cups milk 1 cup plain Greek yogurt

4 tablespoons butter, melted 2 tablespoons apple cider vinegar

> Preheat a waffle iron and grease it.

> In a large bowl, combine together flours, sugar, cocoa powder, baking powder, baking soda and salt. In a different bowl, add egg yolks, milk, yogurt, butter and vinegar and beat until fully combined. In a third bowl add egg whites and beat until stiff peaks form. Add milk mixture into flour mixture and beat until fully combined. Gently put in whipped egg whites.

> Place ¼ cup of the mixture into preheated waffle iron and cook for 5 minutes or until golden brown. Repeat with the remaining mixture.

> Store these waffles in a large airtight container. Place wax papers between the waffles to avoid the sticking. These waffles can be stored in the freezer for up to 3 days.

Servings **4** Per Serving**:** *Calories* **470** *Protein* **17.5g** *Carbohydrates* **67.7g** *Fat* **16.9g**

Veggies & Egg Bowl

2 pound Yukon gold potatoes, scrubbed and cut into 1-inch cubes

1 green bell pepper, seeded and cut into 1-inch cubes

1 onion, cut into 1-inch cubes

1 tablespoon olive oil

Salt and freshly ground black pepper, to taste

12 eggs

4-ounce cheddar cheese, shredded

3 scallions, chopped

1 avocado, peeled, pitted and sliced

> Preheat your oven to 425 degrees F.

> In a large bowl, add potatoes, bell pepper, onions, olive oil, salt and black pepper and toss to coat well. until evenly coated. Transfer vegetable mixture onto 2 baking sheets evenly.

> Roast for 35 minutes, stirring and rotating pans once in the middle way. Remove from your oven and keep to the side to cool completely.

> Meanwhile in a different bowl, add eggs, salt and black pepper and beat until fully smooth. Heat a lightly greased large skillet over medium heat and cook the eggs just cooked through, stirring continuously. Put the scrambled eggs onto a plate and keep aside to cool.

> Divide the potato mixture and eggs into 6 containers evenly and top with cheese and scallions. Cover the containers and freeze for 2-3 days. Reheat in the microwave on High for about 2 minutes before serving.

Servings | **6**   Per Serving: *Calories* | **349**   *Protein* | **18.1g**   *Carbohydrates* | **17.7g**   *Fat* | **24g**

Kale & Egg Bowl

½ cup brown rice

2 tablespoons olive oil

2 garlic cloves, minced

¼ teaspoon red pepper flakes, crushed

4 cups fresh kale, chopped

¼ cup Parmesan cheese, grated

1 avocado, peeled, pitted and sliced

4 hard-boiled eggs

> In a large pan add 1 cup of water and cook rice according to package directions. Remove from heat and keep to the side.

> In a large skillet, heat oil over high heat and sauté garlic and red pepper flakes for 60 seconds. Stir in kale and cook for 6 minutes. Stir in Parmesan and remove from heat.

> Peel the boiled eggs and cut in half lengthwise. Divide rice, kale, avocado and eggs in 4 airtight containers and refrigerate overnight.

Servings **4** Per Serving: *Calories* **497** *Protein* **22.4g** *Carbohydrates* **30.3g** *Fat* **30.8g**

Sausage & Beans Bowl

½ pound mild turkey breakfast sausage, sliced

1 teaspoon butter

6 eggs, beaten

1 cup cooked quinoa

1 (15-ounce) can black beans, rinsed and drained

1 cup chunky salsa

> Heat a non-stick skillet over medium heat and cook sausage until done fully. Put the sausage into a bowl.

> With a paper towel wipe out the skillet. In the same skillet, melt butter over medium heat. Add eggs and cook, for 3 minutes or until completely done, stirring often. Fold in cooked sausage and then remove from heat.

> Divide cooked quinoa in 4 mason jars, followed by black beans, sausage mixture, salsa and cheese. Cover with a lid and preserve in your refrigerator for up to 2 days.

> Reheat in microwave before serving.

Servings **4** Per Serving**:** Calories **832** Protein **49.3g** Carbohydrates **98.1g** Fat **27.8g**

Broccoli Omelet

20-ounce frozen broccoli florets
12 eggs
1 cup half-and-half
¼ teaspoon fresh rosemary, minced
¼ teaspoon ground nutmeg
¼ teaspoon red pepper flakes, crushed
Salt and freshly ground black pepper, to taste
6-ounce sharp cheddar cheese, grated

> Preheat the oven to 350 degrees F. Lightly, grease 8 wide mouth mason jars.

> In a pan of lightly salted boiling water, add broccoli and cook for 60 seconds. Drain fully and pat dry with paper towel. Chop the broccoli florets roughly.

> In a large bowl, add remaining ingredients except cheese and beat until fully combined. Add broccoli and cheese and stir to combine.

> Arrange the jars in a rimmed baking dish. Bake for 40 minutes. Remove from oven and keep onto a wire rack to cool completely. Cover with a lid and preserve in freezer for up to 4 days.

> Thaw the omelet and reheat frozen omelets in microwave before serving.

Servings **8**   Per Serving: *Calories* **237**   *Protein* **15.3g**   *Carbohydrates* **4.7g**   *Fat* **17.1g**

Asparagus Frittata

4-ounce pancetta, chopped

8-ounce thin asparagus stalks, trimmed and cut into ¼-inch pieces

12 large eggs   ¼ cup milk

Salt and freshly ground black pepper, to taste

¾ cup mozzarella cheese, shredded   ¼ cup Parmesan cheese, shredded

2½ tablespoons unsalted butter, melted   ½ cup Italian seasoned breadcrumbs

> Preheat your oven to 375 degrees . Grease 4 (4-ounce) mason jars.

> Heat a non-stick skillet over medium heat and cook pancetta until crispy. Using a slotted spoon put the pancetta in a bowl. Discard the pancetta fat, leaving 1 tablespoon in the skillet.

> In the same skillet, add asparagus and cook for 3 minutes. Remove from heat and keep to the side.

> In a large bowl, add eggs, milk, salt and black pepper and beat until fully combined. Add both cheeses and stir to combine fully. In a different small bowl, mix together butter and breadcrumbs.

> In the bottom of each prepared jar, divide the breadcrumbs mixture evenly. With your hands, gently press the mixture. Put egg mixture over breadcrumbs mixture, followed by asparagus and pancetta evenly.

> Arrange the jars in a baking dish. Bake for 13 minutes. Remove from your oven and keep onto a wire rack to cool completely. Cover with a lid and preserve in refrigerator for up to 4 days.

> Reheat in microwave before serving.

Servings **6**   Per Serving**:**   *Calories* **404**   *Protein* **28.3g**   *Carbohydrates* **10.5g**   *Fat* **27.7g**

Sausage Casserole

1 teaspoon butter

2 sweet Italian sausage links

6 eggs

¼ cup coconut milk

Salt and freshly ground black pepper, to taste

1 small sweet potato, peeled and shredded

1 shallot, chopped finely

> Preheat your oven to 375 degrees F. Grease 2 (16-ounce) mason jars with cooking spray.

> In a large skillet, melt butter over high heat and cook sausage until browned fully, breaking apart. Remove from heat and keep to the side.

> In a large bowl, add eggs, coconut milk, salt and black pepper and beat until fully combined. Add cooked sausage, sweet potato and shallot and stir to combine completely. Divide the mixture into prepared mason jars. Arrange the jars in a baking dish.

> Pour hot water in the baking dish about ½-inch high on jars. Bake for 50 minutes.

> Remove from your oven and keep onto a wire rack to cool completely. Cover with a lid and preserve in your refrigerator for up to 4 days.

> Reheat in microwave before serving.

Servings **2** Per Serving**:** Calories **380** Protein **21.4g** Carbohydrates **16.9g** Fat **26g**

Lunch Recipes

Watermelon Salad

For Vinaigrette: 4 tablespoons sherry vinegar

Salt and freshly ground black pepper, to taste

5 tablespoons extra-virgin olive oil

For Salad: 2 cups cherry tomatoes, halved

¾ cup fresh cilantro leaves, chopped

4 cups seedless watermelon, cubed

½ cup feta cheese, crumbled

> For the vinaigrette: in a bowl, add vinegar, salt and black pepper and beat well. Slowly add oil, beating continuously until a thick dressing forms.

> In the bottom of 2 large mason jars, place dressing evenly. Add the salad ingredients in the layers of tomatoes, followed by cilantro, watermelon and feta.

> Cover each jar with the lid tightly and refrigerate for 24 hours. Shake the jars well just before serving.

Servings **2**   Per Serving: **534**   Calories **74**   Protein **8.8g**   Carbohydrates **31.6g**   Fat **43.8g**

Apple Salad

For Dressing: 4 tablespoons almond butter   2 tablespoons maple syrup

2 tablespoons wine vinegar   4 teaspoons sesame oil, toasted

For Salad: 1 medium green apple, cored and sliced thinly

6 radishes, trimmed and sliced thinly   2 celery stalks, chopped

½ cup pecans, chopped   5 cups fresh mixed greens

> For the dressing: in a bowl, add all ingredients and beat until fully combined.

> In the bottom of 2 large mason jars, place dressing evenly. Add the salad ingredients in the layers of apple, followed by radishes, celery, pecans and greens.

> Cover each jar with the lid tightly and refrigerate for 24 hours. Shake the jars before serving.

Servings **2**   Per Serving: *Calories* **932**   *Protein* **25.5g**   *Carbohydrates* **121.2g**   *Fat* **51,5g**

Pomegranate & Apple Salad

For Dressing: 4 tablespoons sherry vinegar

Salt and freshly ground black pepper, to taste

5 tablespoons extra-virgin olive oil

For Salad: 2 pears, cored and sliced thinly

6 cups fresh baby spinach, divided

1 cup fresh pomegranate seeds

½ cup walnuts, chopped roughly

4-ounce blue cheese, crumbled

> For the dressing: in a bowl, add vinegar, salt and black pepper and beat well. Slowly, add oil, beating continuously until a thick dressing forms.

> In the bottom of 2 large mason jars, place dressing evenly. In each jar, add the salad ingredients in the layers of pear, followed by 2 cups of spinach, pomegranate seeds, ½ cup of spinach, pecans, ½ cup of the spinach and blue cheese.

> Cover each jar with the lid tightly and refrigerate for 24 hours. Shake the jars before serving.

Servings **2**   Per Serving: Calories **881**   Protein **23.5g**   Carbohydrates **40g**   Fat **70.9g**

Berries Salad

For Dressing:
- ¼ cup fresh orange juice
- 2 tablespoons fresh lemon juice
- 2 tablespoons extra-virgin olive oil
- 1 tablespoon honey
- 1 teaspoon fresh lemon zest, grated finely

For Salad:
- 2 cups fresh strawberries, hulled and sliced
- 2 cups fresh blueberries
- 2 cups fresh blackberries
- 1 cup almonds, toasted and chopped

> For the dressing: in a bowl, add all ingredients and beat very well.

> In the bottom of 4 large mason jars, divide the dressing. Divide the salad ingredients in the layers of blackberries, followed by strawberries, blueberries and almonds.

> Cover each jar with the lid tightly and refrigerate for 24 hours. Shake the jars before serving.

Servings **4** Per Serving: Calories **318** Protein **7.3g** Carbohydrates **34.2g** Fat **19.8g**

Mixed Fruit Salad

1 large apple, cored and chopped

1 medium tangerine, peeled and sliced

1 cup fresh pineapple, chopped

1 cup fresh blueberries

2 tablespoons fresh lemon juice

3 tablespoons walnuts, chopped

> In 2 large mason jars, divide the salad ingredients in the layers of apple, followed by the tangerine, pineapple, and blueberries. Drizzle with lemon juice and top with the walnuts.

> Cover each jar with the lid tightly and refrigerate for 24 hours. Shake the jars well just before serving.

Servings **2**   Per Serving**:**   *Calories* **175**   *Protein* **3.7g**   *Carbohydrates* **27.7g**   *Fat* **7.3g**

Tropical Fruit Salad

For Dressing: 2 cups fresh strawberries, hulled   ¼ cup fresh mint leaves
¼ cup honey   2 tablespoons fresh lemon juice

For Salad: 2 cups seedless watermelon, chopped

2 cups pineapple, chopped

1 cup strawberries, hulled and chopped

1 mango, peeled, pitted and chopped

1 cup fresh blueberries

> For dressing: in a food processor, add all ingredients and pulse until full combined.

> In the bottom of 4 large mason jars, divide the dressing. Divide the salad ingredients in the layers of watermelon, followed by pineapple, strawberries, mango and blueberries.

> Cover each jar with the lid tightly and refrigerate for 24 hours. Shake the jars well just before serving.

Servings **4**   Per Serving: *Calories* **238**   *Protein* **2.9g**   *Carbohydrates* **60.8g**   *Fat* **1.1g**

Rainbow Veggie Salad

For Dressing:	1/3 cup grapeseed oil	½ cup fresh lemon juice

1 tablespoon fresh ginger, grated

2 teaspoons whole grain mustard

2 teaspoons pure maple syrup	¼ teaspoon salt

For Salad:	2 avocados, peeled, pitted and chopped

2 tablespoons fresh lemon juice

2 cups fresh baby kale, sliced thinly	2 cups small broccoli florets

1 cup red cabbage, shredded	1 cup purple cabbage, shredded

2 large carrots, peeled and grated

1 small orange bell pepper, seeded and sliced into matchsticks

1 small yellow bell pepper, seeded and sliced into matchsticks

½ cup fresh parsley leaves, chopped

1 cup walnuts, chopped	1 tablespoon sesame seeds

> For the dressing: in a food processor, add all ingredients and pulse until fully combined. Transfer dressing into a small jar and refrigerate for 24 hours.

> Meanwhile, in a bowl, add avocado slices and drizzle with lime juice.

> In 6 containers, divide avocado and remaining vegetable and refrigerate for 24 hours.

> Before serving, drizzle each portion with dressing and serve.

Servings **6**	Per Serving:	*Calories* **341**	*Protein* **8.7g**	*Carbohydrates* **21g**	*Fat* **27.4g**

Zucchini Noodles Salad

6 teaspoons extra-virgin olive oil

2 teaspoons balsamic vinegar

Salt and freshly ground black pepper, to taste

1 large zucchini, spiralized with Blade C

2 cups cooked farro

1 cup fresh mozzarella pearls

2 cups grape tomatoes

¼ cup fresh basil leaves

> In a small bowl, add oil, vinegar, salt and black pepper and beat until fully combined.

> In the bottom of 2 large mason jars, divide the vinaigrette. Divide the salad ingredients in the layers of zucchini, farro, mozzarella, tomatoes and basil.

> Cover each jar with the lid tightly and refrigerate for 24 hours. Shake the jars well just before serving.

Servings **2**   Per Serving: *Calories* **361**   *Protein* **13.8g**   *Carbohydrates* **42.1g**   *Fat* **17.2g**

Zucchini & Cucumber Salad

For Dressing:
- 1 small avocado, peeled, pitted and chopped
- ¼ cup plain yogurt
- 1 shallot, chopped
- 1 garlic clove, chopped
- 2 tablespoons fresh parsley
- 2 tablespoons fresh lemon juice

For Salad:
- ½ cup celery, sliced
- ½ cup red bell pepper, seeded and sliced thinly
- ½ cup red onion, sliced thinly
- ½ cup cucumber, sliced thinly
- 6 cups shredded spinach
- ½ cup cherry tomatoes, halved
- ¼ cup feta cheese, crumbled
- ¼ cup Kalamata olives, pitted
- 2 medium zucchinis, cut into thin slices

> For the dressing: in a food processor, add all ingredients and blend until completely smooth.

> In the bottom of 4 large mason jars, divide the dressing. Divide the salad ingredients in the layers of celery, bell pepper, onion, cucumber, spinach, tomatoes, cheese, olives and zucchini.

> Cover each jar with the lid tightly and refrigerate for 3 days. Shake the jars well just before serving.

Servings **4**   Per Serving**:**   *Calories* **199**   *Protein* **6.7g**   *Carbohydrates* **16.7g**   *Fat* **13.5g**

Tofu & Veggie Salad

For Dressing:
- ½ cup smooth peanut butter
- ¼ cup rice vinegar
- 3 tablespoons soy sauce
- 2 tablespoons water
- 1 teaspoon sesame oil, toasted
- 1 teaspoon Sriracha

For Salad:
- 6-ounce broccoli, chopped
- 6-ounce cabbage, shredded
- 1 small red bell pepper, seeded and julienned
- 1 small yellow bell pepper, seeded and julienned
- 1 pound baked tofu, cubed
- ¼ cup edamame, shelled and cooked
- ¼ cup peanuts, roasted
- ¼ cup fresh cilantro leaves

> For the dressing: in a small bowl, add all ingredients and beat until completely smooth. Transfer into a container and refrigerate for 24 hours.

> In a large container, mix together broccoli, cabbage and bell peppers. Cover and refrigerate for 24 hours.

> Before serving, divide salad onto serving plates. Top with the tofu, edamame, peanuts, and cilantro. Drizzle with dressing and serve.

Servings **4** Per Serving: Calories **416** Protein **24.9g** Carbohydrates **22.5g** Fat **28g**

Quinoa & Kale Salad

For Dressing:
- 2 tablespoons olive oil
- 2 tablespoons fresh lemon juice
- ¼ teaspoon dried oregano
- Salt and freshly ground black pepper, to taste

For Salad:
- 6 cups fresh kale, trimmed and chopped
- 1 cup cooked quinoa
- 1 cup tomato, chopped
- 1 cup cucumber, chopped
- ½ cup chickpeas
- ½ cup feta cheese, crumbled
- ½ cup Kalamata olives
- 4 tablespoons hummus
- 2 tablespoons fresh dill, chopped
- 1 lemon, quartered

> For the dressing: in a large bowl, add all ingredients and beat until fully combined. Add kale and with your massage with dressing.

> In 4 mason jars, divide the salad ingredients in the layers of quinoa, kale, tomatoes, cucumber, chickpeas, feta cheese, olives, hummus, dill and lemon.

> Cover each jar with the lid tightly and refrigerate for 24 hours. Shake the jars well just before serving.

Servings | 4   Per Serving: *Calories* | **468**   *Protein* | **18.7g**   *Carbohydrates* | **61g**   *Fat* | **18.5g**

Barley & Cherries Salad

¼ cup prepared salad dressing

1¼ cups cooked pearl barley

4 cups fresh baby spinach

½ cup red onion, chopped

¼ cup dried sour cherries

¼ cup pecans, toasted and chopped

4 tablespoons blue cheese crumbles

> In the bottom of 2 large mason jars, divide the dressing evenly. Divide the salad ingredients in the layers of barley, followed by spinach, onion, cherries, pecans and blue cheese.

> Cover each jar with the lid tightly and refrigerate for 24 hours. Shake the jars well just before serving.

Servings **2**   Per Serving**:**   *Calories* **760**   *Protein* **19.3g**   *Carbohydrates* **118.5g**   *Fat* **26.4g**

Pasta Salad

1 pound penne pasta

2 garlic cloves, chopped

1/3 cup raw walnuts, chopped

Salt, to taste

1¼ cups feta cheese, crumbled and divided

2 cups fresh basil leaves

1/3 cup Parmesan cheese, grated

¼ cup extra-virgin olive oil

2 cups cherry tomatoes, halved

> In a large pan of lightly salted boiling water, cook pasta and cook according to package instructions. Drain the pasta well, reserving ½ cup of cooking liquid. Return the pasta into the pan.

> Meanwhile, for pesto: in a food processor, add basil, garlic, Parmesan, walnuts and salt and blend until fully combined. While motor is running, add the oil and pulse until completely smooth.

> In the pan of pasta, add pesto and ¼ cup of the cooking liquid and stir to fully combine until a saucy mixture forms. Add tomatoes and 1 cup of feta cheese and stir to combine.

> In 4 jars, place the pasta mixture evenly. Top with remaining feta cheese.

> Cover each jar with the lid tightly and refrigerate for 24 hours. Shake the jars well just before serving.

Servings **4**   Per Serving**:**   *Calories* **727**   *Protein* **30.8g**   *Carbohydrates* **70g**   *Fat* **37.1g**

Shrimp & Orange Salad

¼ cup fresh orange juice

3 tablespoons fresh lemon juice

3 tablespoons shallots, minced

Salt and freshly ground black pepper, to taste

1 pound jumbo shrimp, peeled and deveined

1 avocado, peeled, pitted and cubed

2 oranges, peeled, seeded and sectioned

1 fresh fennel bulb, sliced thinly

4 cups fresh spring mix

> Preheat the grill to medium-high heat. Grease the grill grate.

> For dressing in a bowl, add the orange juice, lemon juice, shallots, salt and black pepper and mix until fully combined.

> Transfer half of the dressing in a large bowl. Add shrimp and coat with the dressing generously. Keep to the side to marinate for 20 minutes.

> Grill the shrimp for 3 minutes on each side. Remove from grill and keep aside to cool completely. In the remaining dressing, add avocado cubes and gently, stir to fully combine.

> Divide avocado mixture in 4 mason jars evenly. Place the remaining ingredients in the layers of orange, followed by fennel, shrimp and spring mix.

> Cover each jar with the lid tightly and refrigerate for 24 hours. Shake the jars before serving.

Servings | 4   Per Serving: Calories | 321   Protein | **29.6g**   Carbohydrates | **25.3g**   Fat | **12.2g**

Tuna & Egg Salad

6 hard-boiled eggs, peeled and chopped

½ teaspoon seasoned salt

1 (5-ounce) can water packed tuna, drained

2 cups fresh baby arugula

2/3 cup mayonnaise

½ cup dill pickle, chopped

> In a large bowl, mix together egg, mayonnaise and seasoned salt.

> Divide egg mixture in 2 mason jars evenly. Place the remaining ingredients in the layers of pickles, tuna and arugula.

> Cover each jar with the lid tightly and refrigerate for 24 hours. Shake the jars before serving.

Servings | **2**   Per Serving: Calories | **74**   Protein | **2g**   Carbohydrates | **1g**   Fat | **6g**

Tuna & Veggie Salad

2 (5-ounce) cans water packed tuna, drained

2 tablespoons mayonnaise

Salt and freshly ground black pepper, to taste

½ cup pickled beet slices

¼ cup Kalamata olives

1 cup sugar snap peas, chopped

1 medium carrot, peeled and shredded

1 apple, cored and chopped

2 cups lettuce, torn

½ cup pumpkin seeds, roasted

> In a large bowl, mix together tuna, mayonnaise, salt and black pepper.

> Divide tuna mixture in 2 mason jars evenly. Place the remaining ingredients in the layers of beets, olives, sugar snap peas, carrots, apples, lettuce and pumpkin seeds.

> Cover each jar with the lid tightly and refrigerate for 1 day. Shake the jars before serving.

Servings **2**   Per Serving: *Calories* **637**   *Protein* **48.7g**   *Carbohydrates* **37.4g**   *Fat* **34.4g**

Crab & Rice Salad

2 cups warm cooked white rice

1 teaspoon white sugar

1 tablespoon rice vinegar

1 tablespoon soy sauce

2 large avocados, peeled, pitted and cubed

2 tablespoons fresh lemon juice

2 cucumbers, peeled, seeded and chopped

4 whole nori sheets, chopped finely

1 cup lump crabmeat, picked over

> In a large bowl, place cooked rice.

> In a small pan, add sugar and vinegar over medium heat and cook until sugar dissolves fully, stirring continuously.

> In the bowl of rice, add sugar mixture and soy sauce and toss to coat well. Keep to the side to cool fully. In a different bowl, add avocado and drizzle with lemon juice evenly.

> In the bottom of 4 large mason jars, divide the salad ingredients in the layers of rice, followed by cucumber, nori sheets, crabmeat and avocado.

> Cover each jar with the lid tightly and refrigerate for 24 hours. Shake the jars before serving.

Servings **4** Per Serving: Calories **592** Protein **1.7g** Carbohydrates **89.6g** Fat **20.6g**

Creamy Apple Soup

3 green apples, peeled, cored and chopped

1 teaspoon jalapeño pepper, seeded and chopped

3¼ cups water, divided   ½ cup coconut cream

> In a food processor, add apples, jalapeño pepper and ¼ cup of the water and blend until fully smooth.

> In a pan, add apple puree, remaining broth and water over medium heat and cook for 10 minutes, stirring often. Stir in coconut cream and immediately, remove from heat.

> Remove from heat and keep aside to cool completely.

> Transfer soup into 4 individual meal prep containers. Cover and store in refrigerator for up to 2 days.

Servings **4**   Per Serving: *Calories* **156**   *Protein* **2g**   *Carbohydrates* **24.8g**   *Fat* **7.5g**

Apple & Spinach Soup

2 green apples, peeled, cored and chopped

1 cup unsweetened almond milk   2 cups fresh baby spinach

2 tablespoons chia seeds   ½ teaspoon ground cinnamon

> In a food processor, add all ingredients and blend until fully smooth.

> Transfer soup into 2 individual meal prep containers. Cover and store in refrigerator for up to 2 days.

Servings **2**   Per Serving: *Calories* **173**   *Protein* **2g**   *Carbohydrates* **36.4g**   *Fat* **4.8g**

Peach Soup

8 ripe peaches, peeled and pitted

2 cups fresh baby spinach

2 teaspoons fresh lemon juice

½ cup water

> In a food processor, add all ingredients and blend until fully smooth.

> Transfer soup into 2 individual meal prep containers. Cover and store in refrigerator for up to 2 days.

Servings **2** Per Serving: *Calories* **244** *Protein* **2g** *Carbohydrates* **57.2g** *Fat* **1.8g**

Cherry Soup

2 cups sour cream

2 cups fresh cherries, pitted

2 tablespoons agave nectar

Pinch of ground cinnamon

2-3 drops vanilla extract

> In a food processor, add all ingredients and blend until fully smooth.

> Transfer soup into 2 individual meal prep containers. Cover and store in refrigerator for up to 2 days.

Servings **2** Per Serving: *Calories* **672** *Protein* **8.8g** *Carbohydrates* **56.2g** *Fat* **48.4g**

Strawberry & Rhubarb Soup

3 cups water

4 cups rhubarb stalk, chopped

1½ cups fresh strawberries, hulled and sliced

1/3 cup fresh mint leaves

4-6 drops liquid stevia

Pinch of salt and freshly ground black pepper

> In a pan, add water and rhubarb and bring to a boil. Cook for 5 minutes or until rhubarb becomes soft. Remove from heat and keep aside to cool slightly. In a food processor, add rhubarb mixture and remaining ingredients and blend until fully smooth.

> Transfer soup into 4 individual meal prep containers. Cover and store in refrigerator for up to 2 days.

Servings **4** Per Serving: Calories **46** Protein **1.7g** Carbohydrates **10.3g** Fat **0.5g**

Mixed Fruit Soup

1 peach, peeled, pitted and chopped

2 cups cantaloupe, peeled and chopped

2 tablespoons fresh lemon juice

1 cup fresh peach juice

> In a food processor, add all ingredients and blend until fully smooth.

> Transfer soup into 3 individual meal prep containers. Cover and store in refrigerator for up to 1-2 days.

Servings **3** Per Serving: Calories **76** Protein **1.5g** Carbohydrates **18g** Fat **0.5g**

Quinoa & Berry Soup

2½ cups fresh blackberries

2½ cups fresh blueberries

6 cups unsweetened almond milk

1 tablespoon raw almonds, chopped

2 cups cooked quinoa

> In a food processor, add all ingredients except quinoa and blend until fully smooth. Transfer the mixture in a large bowl. Add quinoa and stir to combine well.

> Transfer soup into 7 individual meal prep containers. Cover and store in refrigerator for up to 2 days. Reheat soup before serving.

Servings | **7**   Per Serving: *Calories* | **270**   *Protein* | **9g**   *Carbohydrates* | **45.5g**   *Fat* | **6.8g**

Beet Soup

2 cups plain yogurt

4 teaspoons fresh lemon juice

2 cups Beets, trimmed, peeled and chopped

2 tablespoons fresh dill

Salt, to taste

> In a high-speed blender, add all ingredients and blend until fully smooth.

> Transfer soup into 2 individual meal prep containers. Cover and store in refrigerator for up to 2 days. Reheat soup before serving.

Servings | **2**   Per Serving: *Calories* | **259**   *Protein* | **17.5g**   *Carbohydrates* | **36.1g**   *Fat* | **3.5g**

Zucchini Soup

2 cups water

2 teaspoons flax oil

2 cups zucchini, peeled and chopped

2 tablespoons onion, chopped

1 garlic clove, chopped

2 teaspoons curry powder

Salt and freshly ground black pepper, to taste

> In a high-speed blender, add all ingredients and blend until fully smooth.

> Transfer soup into 2 individual meal prep containers. Cover and store in refrigerator for up to 1-2 days. Reheat soup before serving.

Servings | **2**   Per Serving: Calories | **71**   Protein | **1.8g**   Carbohydrates | **6.4g**   Fat | **5.2g**

Split Pea & Kale Soup

2 cups vegetable broth

1 cup cooked split peas

2 cups fresh baby kale

1 small onion, chopped

Salt and freshly ground black pepper, to taste

Pinch of red pepper flakes, crushed

1 teaspoon olive oil

> In a high-speed blender, add all ingredients and blend until fully smooth.

> Transfer soup into 2 individual meal prep containers. Cover and store in refrigerator for up to 2 days. Reheat soup before serving.

Servings | **2**   Per Serving: Calories | **442**   Protein | **3q1.4g**   Carbohydrates | **70.7g**   Fat | **4.9g**

Beans & Artichoke Soup

2 cups water

1 cup cooked white beans

1 cup artichoke hearts

1 cup fresh mustard greens

1 lemon, peeled and seeded

Salt and freshly ground black pepper, to taste

> In a high-speed blender, add all ingredients and blend until fully smooth.

> Transfer soup into 2 individual meal prep containers. Cover and store in refrigerator for up to 1-2 days. Reheat soup before serving.

Servings | **2**   Per Serving**:**   *Calories* | **384**   *Protein* | **27.1g**   *Carbohydrates* | **71.5g**   *Fat* | **1.1g**

Asparagus Soup

1 tablespoon olive oil

3 scallions, chopped

1 garlic clove, minced

1 Serrano pepper, seeded and chopped

1½ pounds fresh asparagus, trimmed and chopped

4 cups vegetable broth

2 tablespoons fresh lemon juice

Salt and freshly ground black pepper, to taste

> In a large soup pan, heat oil over medium heat and sauté scallion for 4 minutes. Add garlic and Serrano pepper and sauté for about 1-2 minutes. Add asparagus and broth and bring to a boil. Reduce the heat to low and simmer, covered for 30 minutes. Remove from heat and keep to the side to cool off.

> In a blender, add soup in batches and blend until fully smooth. Return the soup in pan and cook for 3-4 minutes. Stir in lemon juice, salt and black pepper and remove from heat. Keep to the side to cool fully.

> Transfer soup into 4 individual meal prep containers. Cover and store in refrigerator for up to 1-2 days. Reheat soup before serving.

Servings **4**   Per Serving: *Calories* **109**   *Protein* **8.9g**   *Carbohydrates* **8.9g**   *Fat* **1g**

Broccoli Soup

2 tablespoons olive oil

½ cup onion, chopped

1 garlic clove, minced

1 tablespoon fresh thyme, chopped

2 medium heads broccoli, cut into florets

4 cups vegetable broth, divided

Salt and freshly ground black pepper, to taste

1 avocado, peeled, pitted and chopped

> In a large soup pan, heat oil over medium heat and sauté onion for about 5 minutes. Add garlic and thyme and sauté for 60 seconds. Add broccoli and cook for 5 minutes. Add broth and bring to a boil on high heat. Reduce the heat to medium-low and simmer, covered for about 30-35 minutes. Remove from heat and keep aside to cool slightly.

> In a blender, add soup in batches with avocado and blend until fully smooth. Return the soup in pan and cook for 3-4 minutes. Stir in salt and black pepper and remove from heat. Keep to the side to cool completely.

> Transfer soup into 4 individual meal prep containers. Cover and store in refrigerator for up to 1-2 days. Reheat soup before serving.

Servings **4**   Per Serving: *Calories* **295**   *Protein* **13.1g**   *Carbohydrates* **23.9g**   *Fat* **19.1g**

Cauliflower Soup

2 tablespoons olive oil

1 onion, chopped

2 celery stalks, chopped

2 carrots, peeled and chopped

2 garlic cloves, minced

1½ teaspoons ground cumin

½ teaspoon ground coriander

½ teaspoon paprika

1 head cauliflower, chopped

4 cups chicken broth

1 cup coconut milk

Salt and freshly ground black pepper, to taste

> In a large soup pan, heat oil over medium heat and sauté onion, celery and carrot for about 4-5 minutes. Add garlic and spices and sauté for about 1 minute. Add cauliflower and cook for about 5 minutes, stirring occasionally. Add broth and coconut milk and bring to a boil over medium-high heat. Reduce the heat to low and simmer for about 15 minutes or until desired doneness of vegetables. Remove from heat and keep aside to cool slightly.

> In a blender, add soup in batches and pulse until smooth. Return the soup in pan and cook for 3-4 minutes. Stir in salt and black pepper and remove from heat. Keep aside to cool completely.

> Transfer soup into 4 individual meal prep containers. Cover and store in refrigerator for up to 1-2 days. Reheat soup before serving.

Servings **4** Per Serving: *Calories* **284** *Protein* **8.4g** *Carbohydrates* **14.6g** *Fat* **23g**

Sweet Potato Soup

2 tablespoons olive oil

1 medium onion, chopped

3 large scallions, chopped

2 garlic cloves, minced

1 teaspoon fresh ginger, minced

4 sweet potatoes, peeled and chopped

4 cups chicken broth

1½ cups coconut milk

Salt and freshly ground black pepper, to taste

2 tablespoons fresh lemon juice

> In a large soup pan, heat oil over medium heat and sauté onion for about 4-6 minutes. Add scallions and sauté for about 1-2 minutes. Add garlic and ginger and sauté for about 1 minute. Add sweet potato and cook for about 4-5 minutes. Add broth and bring to a boil over high heat. Reduce the heat to medium-low and simmer for about 10 minutes. Stir in coconut milk and cook for 5 minutes. Season with salt and black pepper and remove from heat. Keep aside to cool slightly.

> In a blender, add soup in batches and pulse until smooth. Return the soup in pan and cook for 3-4 minutes. Stir in lemon juice and remove from heat. Keep aside to cool completely.

> Transfer soup into 6 individual meal prep containers. Cover and store in refrigerator for up to 1-2 days. Reheat soup before serving.

Servings **6**   Per Serving: *Calories* **307**   *Protein* **6.3g**   *Carbohydrates* **28.1g**   *Fat* **20.1g**

Carrot Soup

2½ cups organic coconut water   4 medium carrots, peeled and chopped

1 teaspoon fresh ginger, chopped   ¼ cup raw cashews, chopped

1 teaspoon curry powder   Salt and freshly ground black pepper, to taste

1 tablespoon fresh cilantro, chopped

> In a high-speed blender, add all ingredients except cilantro and pulse until smooth. Transfer the mixture into a soup pan. Cook for about 4-5 minutes or until heated completely.

> Stir in cilantro and remove from heat. Keep aside to cool completely.

> Transfer soup into 2 individual meal prep containers. Cover and store in refrigerator for up to 1-2 days. Reheat soup before serving.

Servings **2**   Per Serving**:**   *Calories* **212**   *Protein* **8.7g**   *Carbohydrates* **30g**   *Fat* **6g**

Peas Soup

3 cups vegetable broth

2 teaspoons curry powder

2 garlic cloves, minced

2 tablespoons fresh mint leaves, chopped

1 (10-ounce) package frozen peas

Salt and freshly ground black pepper, to taste

1 teaspoon olive oil

½ teaspoon cumin seeds

½ teaspoon mustard seeds

> In a large pan, add broth over high heat and bring to a boil. Add curry powder, garlic and mint and stir to combine. Reduce the heat to medium-low and simmer, covered for about 5 minutes. Stir in peas and simmer for about 5 minutes. Remove from heat and keep aside to cool slightly.

> In a large blender, add soup in batches and pulse until smooth. Return the soup into pan on medium heat. Stir in salt and black pepper and cook for about 3-4 minutes.

> Meanwhile, in a small frying pan, heat oil on medium-high heat. Add cumin seeds and mustard seeds and sauté for about 30-45 seconds. Pour oil mixture over soup and keep aside to cool completely.

> Transfer soup into 6 individual meal prep containers. Cover and store in refrigerator for up to 1-2 days. Reheat soup before serving.

Servings **6**   Per Serving**:**   *Calories* **71**   *Protein* **5.3g**   *Carbohydrates* **8.4g**   *Fat* **1.9g**

Spinach Soup

4 cups vegetable broth

10-ounce frozen onion

Salt and freshly ground black pepper, to taste

10-ounce frozen spinach

6 large celery stalks, chopped

> In a large soup pan, add broth and bring to a boil over medium-high heat. Stir in vegetables and again bring to a boil. Reduce the heat to medium and cook for about 5 minutes, stirring occasionally. Reduce the heat to low and simmer for about 10-15 minutes or until desired doneness. Remove from heat and keep aside to cool

> In a large blender, add soup in batches and pulse until smooth. Return the soup into pan on medium heat. Stir in salt and black pepper and cook for about 4-5 minutes. Keep aside to cool completely.

> Transfer soup into 6 individual meal prep containers. Cover and store in refrigerator for up to 1-2 days. Reheat soup before serving.

Servings **6**   Per Serving**:**   *Calories* **58**   *Protein* **5.2g**   *Carbohydrates* **7.2g**   *Fat* **1.2g**

Tomato Soup

2 tablespoons olive oil

2 garlic cloves, minced

½ teaspoon dried thyme, crushed

2 teaspoons balsamic vinegar

¼ cup fresh basil leaves, chopped

Salt and freshly ground black pepper, to taste

1½ cups onion, chopped

2 tablespoons tomato paste

2 cups fresh tomatoes, chopped

4 cups vegetable broth

> In a large soup pan, heat oil over medium heat and sauté onion for about 4-5 minutes. Add garlic, tomato paste and thyme and sauté for about 1 minute. Add tomatoes, vinegar and broth and bring to a boil. Reduce the heat to low and simmer, covered for about 15 minutes. Remove from heat and keep aside to cool slightly.

> In a blender, add soup in batches and pulse until smooth. Return the soup in the pan. Stir in basil and cook for about 3-4 minutes. Season with salt and black pepper and remove from heat. Keep aside to cool completely.

> Transfer soup into 6 individual meal prep containers. Cover and store in refrigerator for up to 1-2 days. Reheat soup before serving.

Servings **6**   Per Serving**:**   *Calories* **95**   *Protein* **4.4g**   *Carbohydrates* **7.1g**   *Fat* **5.8g**

Broccoli & Watercress Soup

1 tablespoon olive oil

1 small onion, chopped

1 garlic clove, minced

1 head broccoli, cut into small florets

2½ cups water

Salt and freshly ground black pepper, to taste

¾ cup watercress

1 tablespoon fresh lemon juice

> In a large soup pan, heat oil over medium heat and sauté onion for about 4-5 minutes. Add garlic and sauté for about 1 minute. Add broccoli and cook for about 4 minutes. Add water and bring to a boil. Reduce the heat to low and simmer, covered for about 8 minutes or until desired doneness. Remove from heat and keep aside to cool slightly.

> In a blender, add soup in batches with arugula and pulse until smooth. Return the soup into pan over medium heat. Stir in salt and black pepper and cook for about 3-4 minutes. Stir in lemon juice and remove from heat. Keep aside to cool completely.

> Transfer soup into 2 individual meal prep containers. Cover and store in refrigerator for up to 1-2 days. Reheat soup before serving.

Servings **2**   Per Serving**:**   *Calories* **183**   *Protein* **8.2g**   *Carbohydrates* **23.9g**   *Fat* **9.3g**

Greens Soup

2 cups collard greens, chopped

2 cups mustard greens, chopped

1 large onion, chopped

2 teaspoons fresh ginger, chopped

2 tablespoons soy sauce

10 cups vegetable broth

Salt and freshly ground black pepper, to taste

> In a large soup pan, add all ingredients and bring to a boil over high heat. Reduce the heat to medium and simmer, covered for about 25-30 minutes. Remove from heat and keep aside to cool slightly.

> In a blender, add soup in batches and pulse until smooth.

> Transfer soup into 8 individual meal prep containers. Cover and store in refrigerator for up to 1-2 days. Reheat soup before serving.

Servings **8**   Per Serving**:**   Calories **66**   Protein **2g**   Carbohydrates **4.8g**   Fat **1.9g**

Mushroom Soup

4 cups fresh cremini mushrooms, rinsed and chopped

2 tablespoons onion, chopped

2 garlic cloves, chopped

1 Serrano pepper, seeded and chopped

1 tablespoon fresh thyme leaves, chopped

¼ teaspoon red pepper flakes, crushed

1 cup coconut milk

2 cups vegetable broth

Salt and freshly ground black pepper, to taste

2 tablespoons arrowroot powder

2 tablespoons fresh lemon juice

> In a high-speed blender add mushrooms and pulse until chopped finely. Add remaining all ingredients except arrowroot powder and lemon juice and pulse until smooth and creamy. Transfer the mixture into a large soup pan over medium heat. Slowly, add arrowroot powder, stirring continuously. Cook for about 5-10 minutes or until desired doneness, stirring occasionally. Stir in lemon juice and immediately remove from heat. Keep aside to cool completely.

> Transfer soup into 4 individual meal prep containers. Cover and store in refrigerator for up to 1-2 days. Reheat soup before serving.

Servings **4**   Per Serving: *Calories* **185**   *Protein* **5.g**   *Carbohydrates* **12.5g**   *Fat* **15.2g**

Pumpkin Soup

1 tablespoon olive oil 1 medium yellow onion, chopped

2 garlic cloves, minced ¼ teaspoon fresh ginger, minced

1 jalapeño pepper, chopped 2 tablespoons fresh cilantro, chopped

3 cups pumpkin, peeled, seeded and cubed 4¼ cups vegetable broth

1 teaspoon fresh lime peel, grated finely

Salt and freshly ground black pepper, to taste ½ cup coconut cream

2 tablespoons fresh lime juice

> In a large soup pan, heat oil over medium heat and sauté onion for about 5-6 minutes. Add garlic, ginger, jalapeño and cilantro and sauté for 1 minute. Add pumpkin and cook for about 4-5 minutes. Add broth and bring to a boil on high heat. Reduce the heat to low and simmer for about 15 minutes. Remove from heat and keep aside to cool slightly.

> In a blender, add soup in batches with coconut cream and pulse until smooth. Return the soup in pan and cook for 4-5 minutes. Stir in time juice and remove from heat. Keep aside to cool completely.

> Transfer soup into 4 individual meal prep containers. Cover and store in refrigerator for up to 1-2 days. Reheat soup before serving.

Servings **4**   Per Serving**:**   *Calories* **217**   *Protein* **8.3g**   *Carbohydrates* **20.9g**   *Fat* **12.7g**

Bell Pepper Soup

1½ cups red bell pepper, seeded and chopped

¾ cup vegetable broth   1/3 cup raw cashews

Salt and freshly ground black pepper, to taste

> In a high-speed blender, add all ingredients and pulse until smooth. Transfer the soup in a pan over medium heat ands simmer for about 3-4 minutes. Remove from heat and keep aside to cool completely.

> Transfer soup into 2 individual meal prep containers. Cover and store in refrigerator for up to 1-2 days. Reheat soup before serving.

Servings **2**   Per Serving**:**   *Calories* **174**   *Protein* **6.2g**   *Carbohydrates* **14.6g**   *Fat* **11.3g**

Green Veggie Soup

¼ cup almonds, soaked for overnight and drained

1 large avocado, peeled, pitted and chopped

2 cups fresh kale, trimmed and chopped

1 small zucchini, chopped

1 celery stalks, chopped

1 small green bell pepper, seeded and chopped

2 tablespoons scallion (green part), chopped

1 garlic clove, chopped

1 jalapeño pepper, chopped

½ cup fresh cilantro leaves

¼ cup fresh parsley leaves

2 tablespoons fresh lemon juice

2 cups vegetable broth

> In a high-speed blender, add all ingredients and pulse in batches until smooth. Transfer the soup into a pan over medium heat and cook for about 4-5 minutes. Remove from heat and keep aside to cool completely.

> Transfer soup into 4 individual meal prep containers. Cover and store in refrigerator for up to 1-2 days. Reheat soup before serving.

Servings **4** Per Serving**:** *Calories* **194** *Protein* **6.7g** *Carbohydrates* **14.1g** *Fat* **13.7g**

Sweet & Spicy Meatballs

For Meatballs:
- 1 pound ground beef
- 1 egg, beaten
- 2 tablespoons Sriracha
- 2 tablespoons tapioca starch
- 1 tablespoon apple cider vinegar
- 1 teaspoon garlic, minced
- ½ teaspoon ground ginger
- Salt and freshly ground black pepper, to taste

For Sauce:
- 1 cup canned crushed tomatoes, drained
- ¼ cup onion, chopped
- 1 tablespoon garlic, minced
- ½ cup ketchup
- 3-4 tablespoons Sriracha
- 2 tablespoons honey
- ½ tablespoons apple cider vinegar
- 1 tablespoon red pepper flakes, crushed
- ¼ teaspoon ground ginger
- Salt and freshly ground black pepper, to taste
- ½ cup canned pineapple, drained and crushed

> Preheat the oven to 450 degrees F. Grease a large baking sheet.

> For meatballs: in a bowl, add all ingredients and mix until well combined. Make golf ball sized meatballs from mixture. Arrange meatballs onto prepared baking sheet in a single layer.

> Bake for about 12-14 minutes.

> Meanwhile, for sauce in a food processor, add all ingredients except pineapple and pulse until smoot. Transfer sauce into a medium pan and bring to a gentle boil. Add baked meatballs and pineapple stir to combine. Reduce heat to low and simmer for about 10 -15 minutes, coating meatballs with sauce occasionally. Remove from heat and keep aside to cool completely.

> In 4 airtight containers, divide meatballs with sauce and refrigerate for about 1-2 days.

> Reheat slightly before serving.

Servings | **4**   Per Serving: Calories | **346**   Protein | **37.4g**   Carbohydrates | **29.2g**   Fat | **8.7g**

Meatballs with Apple Sauce

For Meatballs:
- 1 pound ground chicken
- 1 teaspoon garlic, minced
- 2 tablespoons fresh cilantro leaves, minced
- 1 tablespoon olive oil
- ½ teaspoon ground cumin
- ½ teaspoon red pepper flakes, crushed
- Salt, to taste

For Apple Sauce:
- 3 medium tart apples, peeled, cored and chopped
- ¼ cup golden raisins
- 3 tablespoons pure maple syrup
- 1 tablespoon apple cider vinegar
- 2 tablespoons almond butter
- ¼ cup water
- ¼ teaspoon ground cumin
- Pinch of red pepper flakes, crushed
- Salt, taste

> Preheat the oven to 400 degrees F. Line a large baking sheet with parchment paper.

> For meatballs: in a large bowl, add all ingredients and mix until well combined. Make desired sized balls from mixture. Arrange the meatballs into prepared baking sheet in a single layer.

> Bake for about 15-20 minutes or until done completely.

> Meanwhile, for sauce in a medium pan, mix together all ingredients over medium-high heat and cook, covered for about 6-8 minutes, stirring occasionally. Uncover and cook for 2-3 minutes more or until desired thickness. Remove from heat and keep aside to cool slightly. With a potato masher, mash the apple pieces slightly to form a chunky mixture.

> In 4 airtight containers, divide meatballs with sauce and refrigerate for about 1-2 days.

> Reheat slightly before serving.

Servings **4** Per Serving: Calories **451** Protein **35.4g** Carbohydrates **42.4g** Fat **16.9g**

Meatballs with Yogurt Dip

2 cups plain yogurt

1 cup salsa

1 teaspoon red chili powder

1 teaspoon ground cumin

2 pounds ground turkey

1 cup canned black beans, rinsed and drained

½ cup oat bran

½ cup fresh parsley, chopped

¼ cup egg whites

¼ cup olive oil

> Preheat the oven to 400 degrees F. Lightly, grease a shallow baking dish.

> For dip: in a large bowl, add yogurt, salsa, chili powder and cumin and mix until well combined. Transfer 1½ cups of yogurt dip in a small bowl and reserve in refrigerator for about 1 day.

> In the bowl of remaining dip, add remaining all ingredients and mix until well combined. Make 24 equal sized balls from mixture. Arrange the meatballs into prepared baking dish in a single layer.

> Bake for about 20-25 minutes. Remove from oven and keep aside to cool completely.

> In 8 airtight containers, divide meatballs with sauce and refrigerate for about 1-2 days.

> Reheat slightly before serving.

> Serve meatballs alongside yogurt dip.

Servings **8**   Per Serving: Calories **455**   Protein **42g**   Carbohydrates **28.6g**   Fat **21.3g**

Chicken & Oat Burgers

6-ounce lean ground chicken

6 tablespoons old-fashioned oats

½ cup unsweetened applesauce

4 tsps dehydrated onion flakes, crushed

1 teaspoon chili powder

Salt, to taste

> Preheat the broiler of oven. Grease a broiler pan.

> For burger in a large bowl, add all ingredients and mix until well combined. Make 2 burger from mixture. Arrange the burger onto prepared broiler pan.

> Broil the burger for about 5 minutes per side. Remove from grill and keep aside to cool completely.

> **Store** these burgers in an airtight container, by placing parchment papers between the burgers to avoid the sticking. These burgers can be stored in the freezer for up to 3 weeks.

> Before serving, thaw the burgers and then reheat in microwave.

Servings **2**   Per Serving**:**   *Calories* **164**   *Protein* **18.1g**   *Carbohydrates* **12.1g**   *Fat* **4.9g**

Turkey & Apple Burgers

12-ounce lean ground turkey

½ of apple, peeled, cored and grated

½ of red bell pepper, seeded and chopped finely

¼ cup red onion, minced

2 small garlic cloves, chopped finely

1 tsp fresh ginger, chopped finely

2½ tablespoons fresh cilantro, chopped

2 tablespoons curry paste

1 teaspoon ground cumin

1 teaspoon olive oil

> Preheat the grill to medium heat. Grease the grill grate.

> For burgers in a large bowl, add all ingredients except oil and mix until well combined. Make 4 equal sized burgers from mixture. Brush the burgers with olive oil evenly.

> Grill the burgers for about 5-6 minutes per side. Remove from grill and keep aside to cool completely.

> Store these burgers in an airtight container, by placing parchment papers between the burgers to avoid the sticking. These burgers can be stored in the freezer for up to 3 weeks.

> Before serving, thaw the burgers and then reheat in microwave.

Servings **4**   Per Serving**:**   *Calories* **213**   *Protein* **17.7g**   *Carbohydrates* **9.5g**   *Fat* **2.1g**

Beef & Veggie Burgers

1 pound ground beef	1 carrot, peeled and chopped finely

1 medium raw beetroot, trimmed, peeled and chopped finely

1 small onion, chopped finely	2 serrano peppers, seeded and chopped finely

1 tablespoon fresh cilantro, chopped finely

Salt and freshly ground black pepper, to taste	3 tablespoons olive oil

> In a large bowl, add all ingredients except oil and mix until well combined. Make equal sized 12 patties from mixture.

> In a large non-stick skillet, heat oil on medium heat and cook patties in batches and for about 3-4 minutes per side or until golden brown. Remove from heat and keep aside to cool completely.

> **Store** these burgers in an airtight container, by placing parchment papers between the burgers to avoid the sticking. These burgers can be stored in the freezer for up to 3 weeks.

> Before serving, thaw the burgers and then reheat in microwave.

Servings **6**	Per Serving:	*Calories* **217**	*Protein* **23.5g**	*Carbohydrates* **3.9g**	*Fat* **11.8g**

Salmon Burgers

12-ounces canned salmon

½ cup onion, minced

1 garlic clove, minced

2 tablespoons fresh parsley, chopped

3 egg yolks

½ teaspoon paprika

Salt and freshly ground black pepper, to taste

2 tablespoons olive oil

> Preheat the oven to 350 degrees F. Line a large baking sheet with parchment paper.

> In a large mixing bowl, add all ingredients except oil and mix until well combined. Make equal sized 10 patties from mixture. Place patties onto prepared baking dish evenly.

> Bake for about 15 minutes.

> In a large skillet, heat oil on high heat. Remove salmon burgers from oven and transfer into skillet. Cook for about 1 minute from both sides. Remove from heat and keep aside to cool completely.

> Store these burgers in an airtight container, by placing parchment papers between the burgers to avoid the sticking. These burgers can be stored in the freezer for up to 3 weeks.

> Before serving, thaw the burgers and then reheat in microwave.

Servings **5** Per Serving: Calories **177** Protein **15.1g** Carbohydrates **1.9g** Fat **12.6g**

Beans & Veggie Burgers

½ cup walnuts

1 celery stalk, chopped

5 garlic cloves, chopped

2½ cups sweet potato, peeled and grated

¼ teaspoon cayenne pepper

Salt and freshly ground black pepper, to taste

1 carrot, peeled and chopped

4 scallions, chopped

2¼ cups cooked black beans

½ tsp red pepper flakes, crushed

> Preheat the oven to 400 degrees F. Line a baking sheet with parchment paper.

> In a food processor, add walnuts and pulse until grounded finely. Add carrot, celery, scallion and garlic and pulse until chopped finely. Transfer the vegetable mixture into a large bowl.

> In the same food processor, add beans and pulse until chopped. Add 1½ cups of sweet potato and pulse until a chunky mixture forms. Transfer the bean mixture into the bowl with vegetable mixture. Stir in remaining sweet potato and spices and mix until well combined. Make 8 patties from mixture. Arrange patties onto prepared baking sheet in a single layer.

> Bake for about 25 minutes. Remove from oven and keep aside to cool completely.

> **Store** these burgers in an airtight container, by placing parchment papers between the burgers to avoid the sticking. These burgers can be stored in the freezer for up to 3 weeks.

> Before serving, thaw the burgers and then reheat in microwave.

Servings **4**   Per Serving: *Calories* **600**   *Protein* **30.6g**   *Carbohydrates* **99.6g**   *Fat* **11.1g**

Chicken Pitas

2 (8-ounce) chicken breasts
2 tablespoons olive oil, divided
Salt and freshly ground black pepper, to taste
1 red onion, cut into chunks
1 red bell pepper, seeded and cut into chunks
1 zucchini, cut into chunks
1/3 cup pesto
4 pita pockets

> Preheat the oven to 425 degrees F.

> In a bowl, add chicken breast, 1 tablespoon of oil, salt and black pepper and toss to coat well. Arrange chicken breasts onto a baking dish.

> In another bowl, add vegetables, remaining 1 tablespoon of oil, salt and black pepper and toss to coat well. Arrange vegetables onto another baking dish.

> Arrange both baking dishes in oven. Roast chicken breasts for about 25 minutes, flipping once after 10 minutes. Rost vegetables for about 20-25 minutes, flipping once after 10 minutes.

> Remove from oven and keep both baking dishes aside to cool.

> After cooling, cut chicken breasts into thin strips.

> In a large bowl, add chicken strips, vegetables and pesto and toss to coat well. Divide chicken mixture into 4 airtight containers and refrigerate for about 1-2 days.

> Just before serving, cut the pita in half. Open the pocket and place chicken mixture into each pocket. Serve immediately.

Servings **4**   Per Serving: Calories **559**   Protein **41.5g**   Carbohydrates **41.2g**   Fat **25g**

Chicken & Beans Bowl

½ cup plain Greek yogurt

1 Chipotle pepper in adobo sauce, minced

1 garlic clove, minced

1 tablespoon fresh lime juice

1 cup brown rice

1 tablespoon olive oil

1½ pounds ground chicken

½ teaspoon dried oregano

½ teaspoon ground cumin

½ teaspoon garlic powder

½ teaspoon onion powder

½ teaspoon red chili powder

¼ teaspoon paprika

Salt and freshly ground black pepper, to taste

1 (15-ounce) can black beans, drained and rinsed

1 (15¼-ounces) can whole kernel corn, drained

½ cup Pico de Gallo

> For sauce: in a bowl, add yogurt, chipotle pepper, garlic and lime juice and mix until well combined. Keep aside until using.

> Cook brown rice according to package's instructions. Remove from heat and keep aside.

> In a large Dutch oven, heat oil over medium-high heat and cook ground chicken, oregano, spices, salt and black pepper for about 4-5 minutes. Drain excess grease from pan.

> In the bottom of 6 airtight containers, divide rice, followed by chicken mixture, black beans, corn, Pico de Gallo and top with sauce. Refrigerate for about 1 day.

> Reheat slightly before serving.

Servings | **6**   Per Serving: *Calories* | **889**   *Protein* | **54.3g**   *Carbohydrates* | **145g**   *Fat* | **16g**

Sausage & Beans Bowl

½-pound sliced mild turkey breakfast sausage

1 teaspoon butter

6 eggs, beaten

1 cup cooked quinoa

1 (15-ounce) can black beans, rinsed and drained

1 cup chunky salsa

> Heat a non-stick skillet over medium heat and cook sausage and cook until done completely. Transfer the sausage into a bowl.

> With a paper towel wipe out the skillet. In the same skillet, melt butter over medium heat. Add eggs and cook, for about 2-3 minutes or until done. Fold in cooked sausage and remove from heat.

> Divide cooked quinoa in 4 mason jars, followed by black beans, sausage mixture, salsa and cheese.

> Cover each jar with the lid tightly and refrigerate for about 1 day. Reheat slightly before serving.

Servings **4**   Per Serving: Calories **643**   Protein **38.8g**   Carbohydrates **98.1g**   Fat **11.9g**

Pork & Beans Bowl

For Carnitas:
- 1 pound pork loin
- 1 tablespoon garlic, minced
- 1 tablespoon fresh orange juice
- 1/3 cup fresh lime juice
- 3 teaspoons ground cumin
- 2 teaspoons paprika
- Salt and freshly ground black pepper, to taste
- ¼ cup green chiles

For Corn:
- 1 can yellow sweet corn
- 2 tablespoons fresh lime juice
- 2 tablespoons fresh cilantro, chopped
- 1/3 cup red onion, finely chopped
- 1/3 cup cotija cheese, crumbled
- ½ teaspoon apple cider vinegar
- ½ teaspoon paprika
- Salt and freshly ground black pepper, to taste

For Bowl:
- 8 cups lettuce, torn
- 3 cups cooked brown rice
- 1½ cups black beans, rinsed and drained

> For Carnitas: in a slow cooker, place pork loin and garlic. Set slow cooker on High and cook, covered for about 2-4 hours. Uncover and transfer pork into a large bowl. With 2 forks, shred the meat. Add remaining ingredients and mix well.

> For corn: in another bowl, mix together all ingredients.

> Divide lettuce in 6 containers, followed by pork, brown rice, corn, black beans and cheese. Refrigerate for about 1 day.   Reheat slightly before serving.

Servings 6   Per Serving: Calories 763   Protein 49.5g   Carbohydrates 108.7g   Fat 19.8g

Beans & Rice Burritos

6 warm tortillas

2 cups cooked rice

1 tablespoon olive oil

2 (16-ounce) cans refried beans

½ cup mild salsa

1 cup carrot, peeled and shredded

> Preheat the oven to 375 degrees F.

> In a pan, add beans over medium-low heat and cook until warmed through.

> Place tortillas onto a sooth surface. Place beans in the shape of a log over the center of each tortilla. Top with rice, salsa and carrot. Starting from the edge, tightly wrap each tortilla over the fillings to seal. Tuck the sides in and continue rolling like a burrito. Arrange burrito onto a baking sheet.

> Bake for about 15 minutes, or until light golden. Remove from oven and keep aside to cool completely.

> Transfer the burritos into a container and freeze for 2-3 days. Reheat in microwave for about 1½ minutes before serving.

Servings **6** Per Serving: Calories **452** Protein **14.5g** Carbohydrates **86.3g** Fat **86.3g**

Glazed Shrimp

1/3 cup honey

¼ cup soy sauce

1 tablespoon garlic, minced

1 teaspoon fresh ginger, minced

1 pound medium uncooked shrimp, peeled and deveined[1]

2 teaspoons olive oil

> In a large bowl, add honey, soy sauce, garlic and ginger and beat until well combined.

> Transfer half of sauce into a small jar and refrigerate until using.

> In the bowl, of remaining sauce, add shrimp and toss t coat well. Refrigerate for about 15 minutes.

> Remove shrimp from bowl and discard marinade. In a skillet, heat oil over medium-high heat and cook shrimp for about 1 minute per side. Remove from heat and keep aside to cool completely.

> Transfer the shrimp into 4 containers and refrigerate for about 1-2 days. Reheat in microwave before serving. Serve alongside reserved sauce.

Servings **4**   Per Serving**:**   *Calories* **254**   *Protein* **27.1g**   *Carbohydrates* **27.2g**   *Fat* **4.3g**

Shrimp with Zucchini

2 tablespoons olive oil

2 tablespoons unsalted butter

1 pound medium shrimp, peeled and deveined

1 shallot, minced

4 garlic cloves, minced

¼ teaspoon red pepper flakes, crushed

Salt and freshly ground black pepper, to taste

¼ cup chicken broth

2 tablespoons fresh lemon juice

1 teaspoon fresh lemon zest, grated finely

½ pound zucchini, spiralized with Blade C

2 tablespoons Parmesan cheese, grated

> In a large skillet, heat oil and butter over medium-high heat and cook shrimp, shallot, garlic, red pepper flakes; salt and black pepper and cook for about 2 minutes, stirring occasionally. Stir in broth, lemon juice and lemon zest and bring to a gentle boil. Stir in zucchini noodles and cook for about 1-2 minutes.

> Remove from heat and keep aside to cool completely.

> Transfer the shrimp mixture into 4 containers and refrigerate for about 1-2 days. Reheat in microwave before serving.

Servings **4** Per Serving: Calories **246** Protein **26.2g** Carbohydrates **4.1g** Fat **14.7g**

Prawns with Veggies

2 tablespoons coconut oil

1½ medium onions, sliced

1 tablespoon fresh ginger, chopped finely

3 garlic cloves, chopped finely

2½ teaspoons curry powder

3 medium carrots, peeled and sliced thinly

1 medium red bell pepper, seeded and sliced

1 medium green bell pepper, seeded and sliced

1½ pounds prawns, peeled and deveined

1 cup unsweetened coconut milk

2 tablespoons water

2 tablespoons fresh lime juice

Salt and freshly ground black pepper, to taste

> In a large skillet, heat oil over medium-high heat and sauté onion for about 4-5 minutes. Add ginger, garlic and curry powder and sauté for about 1 minute. Add bell peppers and carrot and sauté for about 3-4 minutes. Add prawns sauté for about 1 minute. Add coconut milk and water and stir to combine. Cook for about 3-4 minutes, stirring occasionally.

> Stir in lime juice, salt and black pepper and remove from heat. Keep aside to cool completely.

> Transfer the prawn mixture into 6 containers and refrigerate for about 1-2 days. Reheat in microwave before serving.

Servings **6** Per Serving: *Calories* **465** *Protein* **45g** *Carbohydrates* **21.2g** *Fat* **24.4g**

Scallops with Asparagus

2 tablespoons coconut oil

¼ cup shallot, chopped

2 garlic cloves, minced

2 tablespoons fresh rosemary, minced

1 pound fresh asparagus, trimmed and cut into 1-inch pieces

2 teaspoons fresh lemon zest, grated finely

1½ pounds baby scallops

Salt and freshly ground black pepper, to taste

2 tablespoons fresh lemon juice

> In a large skillet, heat oil over medium-high heat and sauté shallot for about 2 minutes. Add garlic and rosemary and sauté for about 1 minute. Add asparagus and lemon zest and cook for about 1-2 minutes. Add scallops and stir to combine. immediately, reduce the heat to medium and cook, covered for about 4-5 minutes, stirring occasionally.

> Stir in lemon juice, salt and black pepper and remove from heat. Keep aside to cool completely.

> Transfer the scallop mixture into 4 containers and refrigerate for about 1-2 days. Reheat in microwave before serving.

Servings **4** Per Serving: Calories **248** Protein **31.5g** Carbohydrates **12g** Fat **8.6g**

Curried Potatoes

½ pound potatoes, peeled and cubed into 1½-inh size   1 garlic clove, minced

4 fresh curry leaves   1 teaspoon curry powder

¼ teaspoon cayenne pepper   1 cup coconut cream

½ cup water

> In a pan, mix together all ingredients over medium heat and cook for about 15-20 minutes or until desired doneness of potatoes, stirring occasionally. Remove from heat and discard the curry leaves. Keep aside to cool completely.

> Transfer the potato mixture into 2 containers and refrigerate for about 1-2 days. Reheat in microwave before serving.

Servings **2**   Per Serving: Calories **360**   Protein **8.9g**   Carbohydrates **25.7g**   Fat **28.9g**

Curried Okra

1 tablespoon olive oil

½ teaspoon cumin seeds

¾ pound okra pods, trimmed and cut into 2-inch pieces

½ teaspoon curry powder

½ teaspoon red chili powder

1 teaspoon ground coriander

Salt and freshly ground black pepper, to taste

> In a large skillet, heat oil over medium heat and sauté cumin seeds for about 30 seconds. Add okra and stir fry for about 1-1½ minutes. Reduce the heat to low and simmer, covered for about 6-8 minutes, stirring occasionally. Uncover and increase the heat to medium. Stir in curry powder, red chili and coriander and cook for about 2-3 minutes more. Season with salt and remove from heat. Keep aside to cool completely.

> Transfer the okra mixture into 2 containers and refrigerate for about 1-2 days. Reheat in microwave before serving.

Servings | **2**   Per Serving**:**   *Calories* | **134**   *Protein* | **2.5g**   *Carbohydrates* | **13.6g**   *Fat* | **7.6g**

Cauliflower with Peas

¼ cup water

2 medium fresh tomatoes, chopped

2 tablespoons olive oil

1 small onion, chopped

½ tablespoon fresh ginger, minced

3 garlic cloves, minced

1 jalapeño pepper, seeded and chopped

1 teaspoon ground cumin

2 teaspoons ground coriander

1 teaspoon cayenne pepper

¼ teaspoon ground turmeric

2 cups cauliflower, chopped

1 cup fresh green peas, shelled

Salt and freshly ground black pepper, to taste

½ cup warm water

> In a blender, add ¼ cup of water and tomatoes and pulse until pureed. Keep aside.

> In a large skillet, heat oil over medium heat and sauté onion for about 4-5 minutes. Add ginger, garlic, ginger, jalapeño pepper and spices and sauté for about 1 minute. Add tomato puree, cauliflower and peas and cook, stirring continuously for about 3-4 minutes. Add warm water and bring to a boil. Reduce the heat to medium-low and simmer, covered for about 8-10 minutes or until desired doneness of vegetables. Remove from heat and keep aside to cool completely.

> Transfer the vegetable mixture into 4 containers and refrigerate for about 1-2 days. Reheat in microwave before serving.

Servings **4**   Per Serving: Calories **124**   Protein **3.6g**   Carbohydrates **12.6g**   Fat **7.6g**

Veggies Stir-Fry

1 tablespoon vegetable oil	½ teaspoon fresh ginger, minced
2 garlic cloves, minced	1½ cups broccoli florets
¾ cup carrot, peeled and julienned	1 tablespoon water
6 fresh shiitake mushrooms, sliced	1½ cups snow peas
½ cup water chestnuts, drained and sliced	1 teaspoon cornstarch
3 tablespoons vegetable broth	3 tablespoons soy sauce
Freshly ground black pepper, to taste	

> In a large skillet, heat oil over medium-high heat and sauté ginger and garlic for about 1 minute. Add broccoli, carrot water and stir fry cook for about 2-3 minutes. Add remaining vegetables and cook for about 1-2 minutes.

> Meanwhile in a bowl, mix together cornstarch, broth and soy sauce. Add broth mixture into skillet and cook for about 1-2 minutes. Stir in black pepper and remove from heat. Keep aside to cool completely.

> Transfer the cauliflower mixture into 4 containers and refrigerate for about 1-2 days. Reheat in microwave before serving.

Servings **4**   Per Serving: *Calories* **173**   *Protein* **6.4g**   *Carbohydrates* **30.2g**   *Fat* **4.1g**

Veggies with Apple

For Sauce: 3 small garlic cloves, minced   1 teaspoon fresh ginger, minced

1 tablespoon fresh orange zest, grated finely

½ cup fresh orange juice   1 tablespoon maple syrup

2 tablespoons soy sauce   2 tablespoons white wine vinegar

1 tablespoon fish sauce

For Veggies & Apple: 1 tablespoon olive oil

1 cup carrot, peeled and julienned

1 head broccoli, cut into florets

1 cup red onion, chopped

1 cup celery stalk, chopped

2 apples, cored and sliced

> In a large bowl, add all sauce ingredients and beat until well combined. Keep aside.

> In a large skillet, heat oil on medium-high heat and stir fry carrot and broccoli for about 4-5 minutes. Add celery and onion and stir fry for about 4-5 minutes. Stir in sauce and cook for about 2-3 minutes, stirring occasionally. Stir in apple slices and cook for about 2-3 minutes. Remove from heat and keep aside to cool completely.

> Transfer potato mixture into 4 containers and refrigerate for about 1-2 days. Reheat in microwave before serving.

Servings **4**   Per Serving: Calories **205**   Protein **4.3g**   Carbohydrates **40g**   Fat **4.4g**

Roasted Veggies

2 large zucchinis, sliced	1 large yellow squash, sliced
3 cups fresh broccoli florets	1 pound fresh asparagus, trimmed
2 garlic cloves, minced	1 tablespoon fresh rosemary, minced
1 tablespoon fresh thyme, minced	½ teaspoon ground cumin
½ teaspoon red pepper flakes, crushed	¼ teaspoon cayenne pepper
2 tablespoons olive oil	Salt, to taste

> Preheat the oven to 400 degrees F. Line 2 large baking sheets with aluminum foil.

> In a large bowl, add all ingredients and toss to coat well. Arrange the vegetables mixture into prepared baking sheets in a single layer. Roast for about 35-40 minutes. Remove from oven and keep aside to cool completely.

> Transfer the chickpeas mixture into 4 containers and refrigerate for 2-3 days. Reheat in microwave before serving.

Servings **4**   Per Serving**:**   *Calories* **148**   *Protein* **7.2g**   *Carbohydrates* **17.7g**   *Fat* **8g**

Roasted Chickpeas & Veggies

2 (15-ounce) cans chickpeas, rinsed and drained

1 pound Brussels sprouts, trimmed and halved

4 sweet potatoes, peeled and cubed   2 tablespoons olive oil

1 teaspoon dried basil, crushed   ½ teaspoon garlic powder

Salt, to taste

> Preheat the oven to **425 degrees F. Line a baking sheet with parchment paper.**

> In a large bowl, add all ingredients and toss to coat well. Spread chickpeas mixture onto prepared baking sheet in a single layer.

> Bake for about **30-35 minutes, stirring after every 10 minutes.** Remove from oven and keep aside to cool completely.

> Transfer the chickpeas mixture into 5 containers and refrigerate for 2-3 days. Reheat in microwave before serving.

Servings **5**   Per Serving: *Calories* **814**   *Protein* **37.4g**   *Carbohydrates* **1g**   *Fat* **6g**

Potato with Chickpeas

2 tablespoons olive oil

1 onion, chopped

1 teaspoon fresh ginger, minced

2 garlic cloves, minced

1 tablespoon hot curry powder

1 teaspoon ground cumin

¼ teaspoon ground turmeric

2 large potatoes, scrubbed and cubed

2 (15-ounce) cans diced tomatoes with liquid

2 (15-ounce) cans chickpeas, rinsed and drained

2 cups vegetable broth

Salt and freshly ground black pepper, to taste

> In a large pan, heat oil over medium heat and sauté onion for about 4-5 minutes. Add ginger, garlic, curry powder and spices and sauté for about 1 minute. Add potatoes and cook for about 3-4 minutes. Add remaining ingredients except cilantro and bring to a boil. Reduce the heat to medium-low and simmer, covered for about 15-25 minutes or until desired doneness. Remove from heat and keep aside to cool completely.

> Transfer the chickpeas mixture into 4 containers and freeze for 2-3 days. Reheat in microwave before serving.

Servings **6** Per Serving**:** *Calories* **691** *Protein* **32.7g** *Carbohydrates* **113.6g** *Fat* **14.2g**

Mushroom with Corn

2 tablespoon vegetable oil, divided
2 cups tomatoes, chopped
1 green chili, chopped
1 teaspoon fresh ginger, chopped
¼ cup cashews
2 tablespoons canola oil
½ teaspoon cumin seeds
¼ teaspoon ground coriander
¼ teaspoon ground turmeric
¼ teaspoon red chili powder
1½ cups fresh shiitake mushrooms, sliced
1½ cups fresh button mushrooms, sliced
1 cup frozen corn kernels
1¼ cups water
¼ cup coconut milk

> In a food processor, add tomatoes, green chili, ginger and cashews and pulse until a smooth paste forms.

> In a pan, heat oil over medium heat and sauté cumin seeds for about 1 minute. Add spices and sauté for about 1 minute. Add tomato paste and cook for about 5 minutes. Stir in mushrooms, corn, water and coconut milk and cook for about 10-12 minutes, stirring occasionally. Remove from heat and keep aside to cool completely.

> Divide mushroom mixture into 4 containers and refrigerate for about 1 day. Reheat in microwave before serving.

Servings **4**   Per Serving: Calories **294**   Protein **5.3g**   Carbohydrates **24g**   Fat **22.1g**

Tofu with Brussels Sprout

1 tablespoon vegetable oil, divided

8-ounce extra-firm tofu, drained and cut into 1-inch slices

Salt, to taste

2 garlic cloves, sliced thinly

1/3 cup pecans, toasted and chopped

3 tablespoons brown sugar

¼ cup chopped fresh cilantro

½ pound Brussels sprouts, trimmed and cut into wide ribbons

> In a skillet, heat ½ tablespoon of oil and sauté tofu and a little salt for about 4 minutes or until golden brown. Add garlic and pecans, and sauté for about 1 minute. Add sugar and cook for about 2 minutes. Remove from heat and stir in cilantro. Transfer tofu into a plate and keep aside to cool completely.

> In the same skillet, heat remaining oil and a pinch of salt over medium-high heat and cook Brussels sprouts for about 5 minutes. Remove from heat and keep aside to cool completely.

> Divide tofu and Brussel sprout into 4 containers and refrigerate for about 1 day. Reheat in microwave before serving.

Servings **4**　Per Serving**:**　*Calories* **204**　*Protein* **8.7g**　*Carbohydrates* **14.9g**　*Fat* **14.1g**

Tofu with Veggies

2 tablespoons sugar   ¾ cup water, divided   1/3 cup rice vinegar

2 tablespoons ketchup   2 tablespoons sherry

4 garlic cloves, minced and divided   2 tablespoons jalapeño, minced

1 tablespoon cornstarch   1½ tablespoons low-sodium soy sauce

2 tablespoons canola oil, divided

1 (14-ounce) package extra-firm tofu, drained and cubed

1 red bell pepper, seeded and sliced thinly

2 carrots, peeled and cut into 1/8-inch thick slices

1 (8-ounce) bunch broccolini, cut into ½-inch pieces

> For sauce in a small pan, add sugar, ½ cup of water and vinegar over medium heat and stir until sugar is dissolved completely. Stir in vinegar, sherry, 2 garlic cloves and jalapeño and bring to a boil. Remove from heat and add cornstarch, beating continuously. Stir in soy sauce.

> Meanwhile, in a large cast iron skillet, heat 1 tablespoon of oil over high heat. Add tofu and cook for about 2 minutes per side. Transfer tofu into a plate.

> In the same skillet, heat 1 teaspoon of oil and stir fry bell pepper for about 2 minutes. Add remaining garlic and sauté for about 20 seconds. Transfer bell pepper mixture into plate with tofu.

> In the same skillet, heat remaining oil and stir fry carrot for about 1 minute. Add broccolini and stir fry for about 3 minutes. Add remaining water and cook for about 3 minutes or until all the liquid is absorbed. Stir in tofu mixture and sauce and remove from heat. Keep aside to cool completely.

> Divide tofu and Brussel sprout into 4 containers and refrigerate for about 1 day. Reheat in microwave before serving.

Servings **4**   Per Serving: *Calories* **151**   *Protein* **3.1g**   *Carbohydrates* **22.3g**   *Fat* **13.1g**

Tempeh in Tomato Sauce

½ cup vegetable oil, divided

2 (8-ounce) packages tempeh, cut into ½-inch slices horizontally

1 large onion, chopped

3 garlic cloves, minced

1 teaspoon dried oregano, crushed

1 teaspoon dried thyme, crushed

1 teaspoon red chili powder

1 teaspoon paprika

½ teaspoon red pepper flakes, crushed

1 large green bell pepper, seeded and sliced thinly

1 large orange bell pepper, seeded and sliced thinly

1 (14½-ounce) can diced tomatoes

¼ cup canned tomato paste

1 teaspoon balsamic vinegar

1 tablespoon maple syrup

> Preheat the oven to 350 degrees F.

> In a large bowl, add 2 tablespoons of oil and tempeh slices and toss to coat well.

> In a large skillet, heat ¼ cup of oil over medium-high heat and cook tempeh slices for about 5-7 minutes. Carefully, change the side and cook for about 5-7 minutes. Transfer the cooked tempeh slices into a paper towel lined plate. Keep aside.

> Meanwhile in another nonstock skillet, heat remaining oil over medium-low heat and sauté onion, garlic, herbs and spices for about 8-10 minutes. Add bell peppers and cook for about 10 minutes. Add remaining ingredients and stir until well combined.

> Transfer the tempeh slices in a large casserole dish and top with tomato mixture evenly. With a piece of foil, cover the casserole dish. Bake for about 1 hour. Remove from oven and keep aside to cool completely.

> Transfer the tempeh mixture into 4 containers and refrigerate for about 1-2 days. Reheat in microwave before serving.

Servings **4**   Per Serving: *Calories* **548**   *Protein* **24g**   *Carbohydrates* **31g**   *Fat* **40.3g**

Spicy Quinoa

2 tablespoons vegetable oil
1 cup uncooked quinoa, rinsed
1 green bell pepper, seeded and chopped
1 medium onion, chopped finely
3 garlic cloves, minced
2½ cups water
1 (8-ounce) can tomato sauce
1 teaspoon red chili powder
¼ teaspoon ground cumin
¼ teaspoon garlic powder

> In a large pan, heat oil over medium-high heat and stir fry quinoa, onion, bell pepper and garlic for about 5-10 minutes or until quinoa is toasted lightly. Stir in remaining ingredients and bring to a boil. Reduce the heat to medium-low and simmer, covered for about 30 minutes, stirring occasionally. Remove from heat and keep aside to cool completely.

> Transfer the quinoa mixture into 4 containers and freeze for 2-3 days. Reheat in microwave before serving.

Servings **4** Per Serving: Calories **257** Protein **7.6g** Carbohydrates **36.4g** Fat **9.7g**

Quinoa with Edamame

3½ cups vegetable broth
2 cups uncooked quinoa, rinsed
2½ cups frozen edamame, shelled
1 tablespoon canola oil
2 green bell peppers, seeded and chopped
2 sweet onions, chopped
6 garlic cloves, minced
2 tablespoons fresh ginger, minced
¼ teaspoon red pepper flakes, crushed
¼ cup low-sodium soy sauce
1 tablespoon hot chile paste

> In a large pan, mix together broth and quinoa over medium-high heat and bring to a boil. Stir in edamame and again bring to a boil. Reduce the heat to medium-low and simmer, covered for about 15-20 minutes.

> In a large skillet, heat oil over medium heat and sauté bell peppers and onions for about 4-5 minutes. Add garlic, ginger and red pepper flakes and sauté for about 1 minute. Stir in soy sauce and chile paste and immediately, remove from heat. Add bell pepper mixture into quinoa mixture and gently, stir to combine. Simmer for about 5 minutes, stirring occasionally. Remove from heat and keep aside to cool completely.

> Transfer the quinoa mixture into 8 containers and freeze for 2-3 days. Reheat in microwave before serving.

Servings **8**　Per Serving:　Calories **257**　Protein **7.6g**　Carbohydrates **36.4g**　Fat **9.7g**

Lentils with Tomatoes

For Tomato Puree: 1 cup tomatoes, chopped   1 garlic clove, chopped
1 green chili, chopped   ¼ cup water

For Lentils: 1 cup red lentils   3 cups water
1 tablespoon canola oil   1 small white onion, chopped
½ teaspoon ground cumin   ½ teaspoon cayenne pepper
¼ teaspoon ground turmeric   ¼ cup tomato, chopped

> For tomato paste: in a blender, add all ingredients and pulse until a smooth puree forms. Keep aside.

> In a large pan, add 3 cups of water and lentils over high heat and bring to a boil. Reduce the heat to medium-low and simmer, covered for about 15-20 minutes or until tender enough. Drain the lentils.

> In a large skillet, heat oil over medium heat and sauté onion for about 6-7 minutes. Add spices and sauté for about 1 minute. Add tomato puree and cook about 5-7 minutes, stirring occasionally. Stir in lentils and cook for about 4-5 minutes or until desired doneness. Stir in chopped tomato and immediately remove from heat. Keep aside to cool completely.

> Transfer the lentil mixture into 4 containers and freeze for 2-3 days. Reheat in microwave before serving.

Servings **4**   Per Serving**:**   *Calories* **220**   *Protein* **13.2g**   *Carbohydrates* **33g**   *Fat* **4.3g**

Pumpkin Macaroni

2 cups elbow macaroni
2 tablespoons butter
2 tablespoons all-purpose flour
Pinch of ground nutmeg
Salt and freshly ground black pepper, to taste
1 cup milk
1 cup whipping cream
1 (15-ounce) can pumpkin
1 cup Fontina cheese, shredded
1 tablespoon fresh sage, chopped
½ cup Parmesan cheese, grated
½ cup breadcrumbs
½ cup walnuts, chopped
1 tablespoon olive oil

> Preheat the oven to 350 degrees F. Grease 6 mason jars.

> In a pan of lightly salted boiling water, cook the macaroni according to package's directions. Drain well and return in the pan. Keep aside covered.

> Meanwhile, in another pan, melt butter over medium heat. Add flour, nutmeg, salt and black pepper and stir to combine. Add milk and whipping cream and cook until mixture becomes slightly thick, stirring continuously. Add pumpkin, Fontina cheese and sage and stir until cheese is melted completely. Add cheese sauce in the pan with pasta and gently, stir to combine.

> In a bowl, mix together remaining ingredients. Transfer the macaroni mixture into prepared mason jars evenly. Top with Parmesan mixture evenly. Arrange the jars in a rimmed baking sheet.

> Bake for about 25 minutes. Remove from oven and keep aside to cool completely.

> Cover each jar with the lid tightly and refrigerate for about 1 day. Reheat in microwave before serving.

Servings **6**   Per Serving: Calories **497**   Protein **19.9g**   Carbohydrates **39.7g**   Fat **19.8g**

Dinner Recipes

Cheesy Chicken Salad

For Dressing:
¾ cup fresh basil leaves chopped finely

5 teaspoons Dijon mustard   5 teaspoons balsamic vinegar

Salt and freshly ground black pepper, to taste

5 tablespoons extra-virgin olive oil

For Salad:
½ pound chopped grilled chicken

1 cup seedless green grapes, halved

1 cup seedless red grapes, halved

1/3 cup walnuts, chopped

1/3 cup Asiago cheese, shredded   4 cups fresh baby spinach

> For dressing: in a blender, add all ingredients except oil and pulse until well combined. While the motor is running, slowly add oil and pulse until smooth.

> In the bottom of 4 large mason jars, divide the dressing evenly. Divide the salad ingredients in the layers of chicken, followed by grapes, pecans, cheese and spinach.

> Cover each jar with the lid tightly and refrigerate for about 1 day. Shake the jars well just before serving.

Servings **4**   Per Serving**:**   *Calories* **443**   *Protein* **24.1g**   *Carbohydrates* **12.5g**   *Fat* **35.6g**

Chicken & Cranberry Salad

3 cups cooked chicken, chopped   ½ cup sweetened dried cranberries

1 large yellow bell pepper, seeded and chopped   2 large celery stalks, chopped

¼ of red onion, chopped   1/3 cup sour cream   1/3 cup mayonnaise

Salt and freshly ground black pepper, to taste

1/3 cup almonds, toasted and chopped   4-ounce feta cheese, crumbled

> In a large bowl, add all ingredients except almonds and cheese and mix until well combined.

> In 4 containers, divide salad evenly and refrigerate for about 1 day.

> Top with almonds and cheese just before serving.

Servings **4**   Per Serving**:**   *Calories* **418**   *Protein* **37.4g**   *Carbohydrates* **12.8g**   *Fat* **23.8g**

Chicken & Fruit Salad

For Salad:
2 cups cooked chicken, chopped
1 large apple, cored and chopped
1 cup seedless red grapes, halved   ¼ cup golden raisins
2 celery stalks, chopped   2 tablespoon fresh lemon juice
½ cup walnut, toasted and chopped

For Dressing:
¾ cup fat-free plain Greek yogurt   ¼ cup fresh orange juice
¼ cup mayonnaise   Salt, to taste

> In a large bowl, mix together all salad ingredients except walnuts. In another bowl, add all dressing ingredients and mix until well combined. Pour dressing over salad and stir to combine.

> In 4 containers, divide salad evenly and refrigerate for about 1 day.

> Top with walnuts just before serving.

Servings **4**   Per Serving: *Calories* **374**   *Protein* **27.6g**   *Carbohydrates* **29.1g**   *Fat* **17.1g**

Chicken & Faro Salad

For Sauce:
- 1 cup whole milk Greek yogurt
- ½ cucumber, grated and squeezed
- 2 tablespoons olive oil
- 1 tablespoon white vinegar
- 1 tablespoon fresh dill, minced
- ½ teaspoon garlic powder
- ¼ teaspoon salt

For Seasoning:
- ¾ tablespoon Italian seasoning
- ½ teaspoon corn starch
- 1 teaspoon garlic powder
- ½ teaspoon onion powder
- ½ teaspoon paprika
- ¼ teaspoon ground cinnamon
- ¼ teaspoon ground nutmeg
- Salt and freshly ground black pepper, to taste

For Salad:
- 4 (4-ounce) boneless, skinless chicken breasts
- 2 tablespoons olive oil, divided
- 1 cup dried farro
- 20 cherry tomatoes, quartered
- 1 cucumber, chopped
- 1½ cups black olives, pitted and chopped
- 1 red onion, chopped
- 1 tablespoon red wine vinegar
- 2 tablespoons fresh lemon juice
- Salt and freshly ground black pepper, to taste

> Preheat the oven to 450 degrees. Line a baking sheet with a greased parchment paper.

> For sauce: in a medium bowl, add all ingredients and stir to combine. Transfer sauce into a small jar and refrigerate for about 1 day.

> For seasoning: in a bowl, mix together all ingredients.

\> Season chicken breasts with seasoning and coat with 1 tablespoon of oil.

\> Arrange chicken breasts onto prepared baking sheet and bake for about 15-20 minutes, or until done completely.

\> Meanwhile, cook your farro according to package's directions.

\> For salad: in a bowl, add remaining ingredients and toss to coat well.

\> In 4 containers, divide farro, followed by chicken breast, salad and top with sauce evenly. Refrigerate for about 3-4 days.

Servings **4**   Per Serving**:**   *Calories* **786**   *Protein* **44.3g**   *Carbohydrates* **56.1g**   *Fat* **46.3g**

Chicken & Chickpeas Salad

1 (9-ounce) package cooked and chopped frozen chicken, thawed

3 cups fresh spinach, chopped

1 (15-ounce) can chickpeas, drained

4 small scallions, chopped

1 small cucumber, seeded and chopped

¼ cup fresh mint, chopped

2 garlic cloves, minced

½ cup plain yogurt

1/3 cup feta cheese, crumbled

Salt, to taste

> In a large bowl, add all ingredients and mix until well combined.

> In 4 containers, divide salad evenly and refrigerate for about 1 day.

Servings **4** Per Serving: *Calories* **561** *Protein* **44g** *Carbohydrates* **72.1g** *Fat* **11.6g**

Turkey & Pasta Salad

For Dressing:
- ½ cup cider vinegar
- 1 cup vegetable oil
- ¼ cup Dijon mustard
- ¼ cup honey

For Salad:
- 12-ounce dried tri-colored spiral pasta
- 3 cups cooked boneless turkey breast, cubed
- 3 cups small broccoli florets
- ½ cup sweet red pepper, seeded and chopped
- ½ cup scallion, chopped

> In a bowl, add all dressing ingredients and beat until well combined. Keep aside.

> In a large pan of salted boiling water, add pasta and cook for about 8-10 minutes or according to package's directions. Drain well. Transfer the pasta into a large bowl and keep aside to cool slightly. Add ½ cup of dressing in warm pasta and stir to combine.

> In another bowl, mix together remaining dressing, turkey and vegetables.

> In 12 containers, divide pasta and turkey mixture evenly and refrigerate for about 1 day.

Servings **12**   Per Serving: *Calories* **339**   *Protein* **14.5g**   *Carbohydrates* **23.9g**   *Fat* **20.9g**

Ground Turkey Salad

1 tablespoon canola oil

2 tablespoons brown sugar

¼ cup water

4 cups cabbage, shredded

2 tablespoons fresh lime juice

1 pound ground turkey

2 tablespoons fish sauce

½ of English cucumber, chopped

½ cup fresh mint leaves, chopped

½ cup peanuts, chopped

> In a large skillet, heat oil over medium-high heat and cook turkey for about 5-6 minutes. Stir in brown sugar, fish sauce and water and cook for about 3-4 minutes or until almost all the liquid is evaporated. Transfer turkey into a bowl and keep aside to cool.

> In a large bowl, mix together remaining ingredients.

> In 4 containers, divide turkey and salad evenly and refrigerate for about 1 day.

Servings **4**   Per Serving**:**   *Calories* **404**   *Protein* **37.7g**   *Carbohydrates* **14.1g**   *Fat* **25.1g**

Turkey & Chickpeas Salad

For Dressing:
- 2 garlic cloves, minced
- 2/3 cup olive oil
- 3 tablespoons balsamic vinegar
- 1 tbsp Dijon mustard
- 1 tablespoon Italian dressing
- Salt and freshly ground black pepper, to taste

For Salad:
- 3 cups cooked turkey, chopped
- 1/3 pound sliced prosciutto, chopped
- 1 (15-ounce) can chickpeas, drained
- 1 cup canned sliced and pitted ripe olives, drained
- 6 medium plum tomatoes, chopped
- 6 cups iceberg lettuce, torn
- ½ cup fresh basil, chopped
- ½ cup fresh scallion, chopped
- 8-ounce deli-sliced Swiss cheese, chopped

> In a bowl, add all dressing ingredients and beat until well combined. Cover and refrigerate to chill before serving. In another large bowl, mix together all salad ingredients. Pour dressing over salad and stir to combine.

> In 12 containers, divide salad evenly and refrigerate for about 1 day.

Servings **12**   Per Serving**:**   *Calories* **413**   *Protein* **26g**   *Carbohydrates* **28.1g**   *Fat* **22.1g**

Steak Salad

For Salad:
- 1 tablespoon soy sauce
- 1 tsp Montreal steak seasoning
- 1 (12-ounce) rib-eye steak
- 2 medium carrots, peeled and grated
- 2 medium English cucumbers, cubed
- 1 large tomato, chopped
- ¼ cup red onion, chopped
- 2 cups romaine lettuce leaves, torn

For Dressing:
- 2 tablespoons olive oil
- ½ teaspoon sesame oil
- 2 tablespoons rice vinegar
- 1 tbsp fresh lemon juice
- 2 tablespoons white sugar
- ¼ teaspoon garlic powder
- 2 pinches red pepper flakes, crushed

> For steak: in a large bowl, mix together soy sauce and steak seasoning. Add beef steak and coat with seasoning mixture evenly. Cover and refrigerate to marinate for at least 1 hour.

> Preheat the grill to medium-high heat. Grease the grill grate.

> Grill the steak for about 6 minutes per side. Remove from grill and place the steak onto a cutting board. Keep aside for about 10 minutes before slicing. With a sharp knife, cut the beef steak diagonally into slices across grain. Keep aside to cool completely.

> In a large bowl, mix together remaining salad ingredients. In another bowl, add all dressing ingredients and beat until well combined. Pour dressing over salad and gently toss to coat well.

> In 3 containers, divide salad and steak slices. Refrigerate for about 1 day.

Servings **3**   Per Serving: Calories **436**   Protein **33.5g**   Carbohydrates **24.2g**   Fat **22.6g**

Ground Beef Salad

- ½ pound extra lean ground beef
- ½ cup ketchup
- 2/3 cup Thousand Island dressing
- 3 dill pickle spears, chopped
- 1 cup cheddar cheese, shredded
- ¼ cup white onion, chopped finely
- 1 tablespoon yellow mustard
- ½ cup cherry tomatoes, halved
- 1 small red onion, sliced thinly
- 2 cups romaine lettuce, chopped

> Heat a non-stick skillet over medium heat and cook beef for about 5-6 minutes. Add ¼ cup of finely chopped onion, ketchup and mustard and stir to combine. Reduce heat to medium-low and cook until for about 3-4 minutes. remove from heat and keep aside and cool.

> In the bottom of 2 large mason jars, divide the dressing evenly. Divide the salad ingredients in the layers of tomatoes, pickles, onions, cheese, beef mixture and lettuce.

> Cover each jar with the lid tightly and refrigerate for up to 4 days. Shake the jars well just before serving.

Servings **2**   Per Serving: *Calories* **847**   *Protein* **47.9g**   *Carbohydrates* **40.5g**   *Fat* **56.3g**

Pork & Grapes Salad

For Dressing: ¼ cup extra-virgin olive oil   2 tablespoons balsamic vinegar   1 medium, shallot, chopped finely   1 tsp fresh thyme, minced   Salt and freshly ground black pepper, to taste

For Pork Chops: 4 (5-ounce) boneless pork chops   1 tsp fresh thyme, minced   Salt and freshly ground black pepper, to taste

For Salad: 4 cups baby arugula   1 cup seedless red grapes, halved   ½ cup blue cheese, crumbled

> Preheat the grill to medium-high heat. Grease the grill grate.

> In a bowl, add all dressing ingredients ad beat until well combined.

> In a large bowl, add pork chops, thyme, 3 tablespoons of dressing, salt and black pepper and combine well. Keep aside for at least 5-10 minutes.

> Grill the chops for about 4-5 minutes from both sides. Remove from grill and keep aside to cool completely.

> In a large bowl, mix together arugula and grapes. Pour remaining dressing over salad and gently toss to coat well.

> In 4 containers, divide salad, pork chops and blue cheese. Refrigerate for about 1 day.

Servings **4**   Per Serving: Calories **396**   Protein **41.5g**   Carbohydrates **6.1g**   Fat **22.7g**

Pork & Veggie Salad

3 tablespoons vegetable oil

1¼ pounds pork tenderloin, sliced thinly

Salt and freshly ground black pepper, to taste

2 carrots, peeled and grated

5 cups Napa cabbage, shredded

2 scallions, chopped

2 teaspoons fish sauce

2 tablespoons fresh lime juice

> In a large skillet, heat oil over medium heat and cook pork with salt and black pepper for about 2 minutes per side.

> In a large bowl, mix together pork and remaining ingredients and toss to coat well.

> In 4 containers, divide salad and refrigerate for about 1 day.

Servings **4**   Per Serving: *Calories* **321**   *Protein* **39g**   *Carbohydrates* **5.6g**   *Fat* **15.4g**

Meat & Veggie Salad

For Dressing:
- 1 tablespoon mayonnaise
- 1 tablespoon buttermilk
- 1 tablespoon plain yogurt
- 1 teaspoon white vinegar
- 1 teaspoon Dijon mustard
- 1 tablespoon blue cheese, crumbled
- Salt and freshly ground black pepper, to taste

For Salad:
- 1 avocado, peeled, pitted and cubed
- 2 teaspoons fresh lime juice
- 4 tablespoons cucumber, chopped
- 4 tablespoons tomato, chopped
- 4 tablespoons red onion, chopped
- 2-ounce low-sodium deli ham, chopped
- 2-ounce low-sodium deli turkey, chopped
- 3 hard-boiled eggs, peeled and chopped
- 2 cooked bacon slices, crumbled
- 2 tablespoons blue cheese, crumbled
- 4 cups romaine lettuce, chopped

> for dressing: in a bowl, add all ingredients and beat until well combined.

> In a bowl, add avocado and lime juice and toss to coat well.

> In the bottom of 2 large mason jars, divide the dressing evenly. Divide the salad ingredients in the layers of cucumber, tomato, onion, ham, turkey, egg, bacon, avocado, blue cheese and lettuce.

> Cover each jar with the lid tightly and refrigerate for about 1 day. Shake the jars well just before serving. Servings **2**   Per Serving: *Calories* **652**   *Protein* **37.9g**   *Carbohydrates* **20.5g**   *Fat* **47.8g**

Shrimp & Veggie Salad

For Dressing: 2 tablespoons natural almond butter 1 garlic clove, crushed
1 tablespoon fresh cilantro, chopped 1 tablespoon fresh lime juice
1 tablespoon maple syrup 2 teaspoons rice vinegar
1 teaspoon sesame oil ½ teaspoon cayenne pepper
¼ teaspoon salt 1 tablespoon water
1/3 cup extra-virgin olive oil

For Salad: 1 pound shrimp, peeled and deveined
Salt and freshly ground black pepper, to taste
1 teaspoon olive oil 1 cup mung bean sprouts
1 cup carrots, peeled and julienned
1 cup red cabbage, shredded 1 cup cucumber, julienned
4 cups fresh baby arugula ¼ cup fresh basil, chopped
¼ cup fresh cilantro, chopped 4 cups lettuce, torn
½ cup almonds, chopped

> For dressing: in a bowl, add all ingredients except oil and beat until well combined. Slowly, add oil, beating continuously until smooth.

> For salad: in a bowl, add shrimp, salt, black pepper and oil and toss to coat well. Heat a skillet over medium-high heat and cook shrimp for about 2 minutes per side. Remove from heat and keep aside to cool.

> Divide dressing in 6 large mason jars evenly. Place the remaining ingredients in the layers of bean sprouts, followed by carrots, cabbage, cucumber, arugula, basil, cilantro, shrimp, lettuce and almonds.

> Cover each jar with the lid tightly and refrigerate for about 1 day. Shake the jars well just before serving.

Servings **6**   Per Serving: *Calories* **313**   *Protein* **22.3g**   *Carbohydrates* **12.4g**   *Fat* **20.6g**

Grains & Mango Salad

For Dressing:
- ¼ cup fresh lime juice
- 2 tablespoons honey
- 1 tablespoon Dijon mustard
- 1 teaspoon white sugar
- ½ teaspoon ground cumin
- 1 teaspoon garlic powder
- Salt and freshly ground black pepper, to taste
- ½ cup extra-virgin olive oil

For Salad:
- 2 cups fresh mango, peeled, pitted and cubed
- 2 tablespoon fresh lime juice, divided
- 2 avocados, peeled, pitted and cubed
- Pinch of salt
- 1 cup cooked quinoa
- 2 (14-ounce) cans black beans, rinsed and drained
- 1 (15¼-ounce) can corn, rinsed and drained
- 1 small onion, chopped
- 1 jalapeño, seeded and chopped finely
- ½ cup fresh cilantro, chopped
- 6 cups romaine lettuce, shredded

> For dressing: in a blender, add all ingredients except oil and pulse until well combined. While the motor is running, slowly add oil and pulse until smooth.

> In a bowl, add mango and drizzle with 1 tablespoon of lime juice evenly. In another bowl, add avocado and sprinkle with a pinch of salt and then drizzle with remaining lime juice evenly.

> In the bottom of 6 large mason jars, divide the dressing evenly. Divide the salad ingredients in the layers of quinoa, followed by mango, black beans, corns, avocado, onion, jalapeño, cilantro and lettuce.

> Cover each jar with the lid tightly and refrigerate for about 1 day. Shake the jars well just before serving.

Servings **6** Per Serving**:** Calories **1248** Protein **47.7g** Carbohydrates **198.6g** Fat **38.5g**

Grains & Sweet Potato Salad

For Salad: 2 small sweet potatoes, peeled and cubed   2 tbsps olive oil

Salt and freshly ground black pepper, to taste

½ cup quinoa   1 cup water

1 cup canned black beans, rinsed and drained

1 green bell pepper, seeded and chopped

4 cups fresh mixed greens

2 tablespoons dried cranberries

1 tablespoon sunflower seeds

For Dressing: ½ cup frozen mango, peeled, pitted and chopped

3 tablespoons water   2 tablespoons balsamic vinegar

> Preheat the oven to 400 degrees F.

> In a bowl, add sweet potato, oil, salt and black pepper and toss to coat well. Transfer the sweet potato mixture in a roasting pan.

> Roast for about 20 minutes, stirring twice. Remove from oven and keep aside to cool completely.

> Meanwhile, in a pan add quinoa and water over medium-high heat and bring to a boil. Reduce the heat to low and simmer, covered for about 15-20 minutes or until all the water is absorbed. Remove from heat and keep aside to cool completely.

> For dressing in a blender, add all ingredients and pulse until a smooth puree forms.

> In the bottom of 2 large mason jars, place the salad ingredients in the layers of beans, followed by quinoa, dressing, red pepper, greens, sweet potato, cranberries and sunflower seeds.

> Cover each jar with the lid tightly and refrigerate for about 1 day. Shake the jars well just before serving.

Servings **2**   Per Serving: Calories **1045**   Protein **40.4g**   Carbohydrates **180.6g**   Fat **19.8g**

Chickpeas & Veggie Salad

For Dressing:
- 1 garlic clove, minced
- 1/3 cup extra-virgin olive oil
- 2 tablespoons fresh lemon juice
- 1 teaspoon red wine vinegar
- ¼ teaspoon dried oregano
- ¼ teaspoon dried parsley
- Salt and freshly ground black pepper, to taste

For Salad:
- 1 small cucumber, peeled, seeded and cubed
- 1/3 cup Kalamata olives, pitted and halved
- 1 (15¼-ounce) can chickpeas, rinsed, drained and patted dry
- 1 small onion, sliced thinly
- ½ cup feta cheese, crumbled
- 1 cup grape tomatoes, halved
- 3 tablespoons pine nuts
- 5 cups romaine lettuce, torn
- 2 cups fresh baby spinach, torn

> For dressing: in a bowl, add all dressing ingredients and beat until using.

> In the bottom of 3 mason jars, divide the dressing. Add the salad ingredients in the layers of cucumber, followed by olives, chickpeas, onion, feta, tomatoes, pine nuts, lettuce and spinach.

> Cover each jar with the lid tightly and refrigerate for about 1 day. Shake the jars well just before serving.

Servings **3** Per Serving**:** Calories **902** Protein **35g** Carbohydrates **102.5g** Fat **43.2g**

Chickpeas & Lentil Salad

1½ cups water   ½ cup dry lentils   ½ (15-ounce) can chickpeas, drained

1 green bell pepper, seeded and chopped

1 red bell pepper, seeded and chopped

1 yellow bell pepper, seeded and chopped   2 tomatoes, chopped

4 scallions, chopped   2 jalapeño peppers, minced   2 tablespoon olive oil

2 tablespoons fresh lime juice   Salt, to taste   ¼ cup fresh cilantro, chopped

> In a large pan, add water and lentils over high heat and bring to a boil. Reduce the heat to low, simmer, covered for about 30 minutes or until all the liquid is absorbed and lentils become tender.

> Transfer the lentils into a large bowl. Add remaining all ingredients and toss to coat well. Keep aside to cool completely.

> In 5 containers, divide salad evenly and refrigerate for about 1 day.

Servings | **5**   Per Serving: *Calories* | **309**   *Protein* | **14.6g**   *Carbohydrates* | **46g**   *Fat* | **8.8g**

Beans & Mango Salad

For Salad: 1 (15½-ounce) can black beans, drained

                      1 cup jicama, pitted and chopped

                      1 cup mango, peeled, pitted and chopped

                      ¼ cup red onion, sliced thinly

For Vinaigrette: 2 tablespoons cider vinegar

                      ¼ cup extra-virgin olive oil

                      Salt and freshly ground black pepper, to taste

> For salad: in a large bowl, mix together all ingredients and mix. In another bowl, add all vinaigrette ingredients and beat until well combined. Pour vinaigrette over salad and gently toss to coat well.

> Divide salad into 4 airtight containers and refrigerate for1 -2 days.

Servings **4** Per Serving**:** *Calories* **150** *Protein* **7g** *Carbohydrates* **22.3g** *Fat* **4.1g**

Beans & Corn Salad

For Salad:
- 1 (10-ounce) package frozen corn kernels, thawed
- 1 (15-ounce) can black beans, rinsed and drained
- 1 (15-ounce) can kidney beans, rinsed and drained
- 1 (15-ounce) can cannellini beans, rinsed and drained
- 1 small green bell pepper, seeded and chopped
- 1 small red bell pepper, seeded and chopped
- 1 small orange bell pepper, seeded and chopped
- 1 red onion, chopped

For Dressing:
- ¼ cup fresh cilantro, minced
- 1 garlic clove, minced
- 2 tablespoons white sugar
- ½ cup red wine vinegar
- ½ cup olive oil
- 1 tablespoons fresh lime juice
- 1 tablespoon fresh lemon juice
- Drop of hot pepper sauce
- ½ teaspoon red pepper flakes, crushed
- Salt and freshly ground black pepper, to taste

> For salad: in a large bowl, mix together all salad ingredients. In another bowl, add all dressing ingredients and beat until well combined. Pour dressing over salad and gently toss to coat well.

> Divide salad into 8 airtight containers and refrigerate for 1-2 days.

Servings | 8   Per Serving: *Calories* | **710**   *Protein* | **37.6g**   *Carbohydrates* | **112.5g**   *Fat* | **14.8g**

Couscous & Beans Salad

For Salad:
- 1 garlic clove, minced
- 2 tablespoons shallots, minced
- 2 teaspoons fresh lemon zest, grated finely
- ¼ cup fresh lemon juice
- 2 tablespoons extra-virgin olive oil
- Salt and freshly ground black pepper, to taste

For Dressing:
- 1 cup cucumber, chopped
- 2 cups canned garbanzo beans, rinsed and drained
- 1 cup plum tomato, chopped
- 1 cup canned cannellini beans, rinsed and drained
- 2 cups canned black beans, rinsed and drained
- 1 cup cooked couscous
- 1 cup goat cheese, crumbled

> For dressing: in a bowl, add all ingredients and beat until well combined.

> In the bottom of 4 large mason jars, divide the dressing evenly. Divide the salad ingredients in the layers of cucumber, followed by garbanzo beans, tomato cannellini beans, black beans, couscous and cheese.

> Cover each jar with the lid tightly and refrigerate for about 1 day. Shake the jars well just before serving.

Servings | 4   Per Serving: Calories | 1216   Protein | 65.9g   Carbohydrates | 187.1g   Fat | 25.2g

Quinoa & Chickpeas Salad

For Dressing: ¼ cup tahini 3 garlic cloves, chopped
1 teaspoon harissa paste 2 tablespoons fresh lime juice
Salt and freshly ground black pepper, to taste ¼ cup water

For Salad: 1 tablespoon coconut oil 1 cup cooked chickpeas
1 medium avocado, peeled, pitted and slice
1 tablespoon fresh lime juice
½ cup cooked quinoa
1 cup carrot, peeled and shredded
½ cup purple cabbage, chopped 4 cups fresh spinach

> For dressing: in a food processor, add all ingredients and pulse until smooth. Transfer dressing into a small jar and refrigerate for 1 day.

> For salad: in a pan, melt coconut oil over medium-high heat and cook chickpeas for about 15 minutes or until crisp. Remove from heat and keep aside to cool completely.

> Meanwhile, in a bowl, add avocado slices and drizzle with lime juice.

> In 3 containers, divide chickpeas, quinoa, avocado, carrot, cabbage and spinach. Refrigerate for 1 day.

> Before serving, drizzle each portion with dressing and serve.

Servings **3** Per Serving: Calories **680** Protein **23.4g** Carbohydrates **76.1g** Fat **34.6g**

Quinoa & Veggies Salad

For Dressing: 1 avocado, peeled, pitted and chopped roughly

4 tablespoons coconut milk   2 tablespoons fresh lime juice

For Salad: ¾ cup cooked quinoa   4 teaspoons fresh cilantro, minced

3 teaspoons coconut flakes

6 asparagus stalks, cut into -inch pieces   ½ cup green peas

2 medium zucchinis, spiralized with Blade C   5 scallions, chopped

½ cup feta cheese, cubed

> For dressing: in a food processor, add all ingredients and pulse until creamy.

> In a bowl, add quinoa, cilantro and coconut flakes and toss to coat.

> In a pan of boiling water, add asparagus and cook for about 1 minute. Add peas and cook for about 3-4 minutes. Through a colander, drain vegetables and keep aside to cool.

> In the bottom of 2 large mason jars, divide the dressing. Divide the salad ingredients in the layers of zucchini noodles, followed by quinoa, scallions, asparagus, peas and feta.

> Cover each jar with the lid tightly and refrigerate for about 1 day. Shake the jars well just before serving.

Servings **2**   Per Serving: *Calories* **677**   *Protein* **22.1g**   *Carbohydrates* **70g**   *Fat* **38g**

Wheat Berries Salad

3 cups water   1 cup soft white wheat berries   Salt, to taste

1½ pounds eggplants, cut into 1-inch slices

1/3 cup extra-virgin olive oil, divided   1½ pounds firm tomatoes, cored

1 serrano chile, seeded and chopped finely   3 garlic cloves, chopped

2 teaspoons ground coriander   2 teaspoons ground cumin

2 tablespoons fresh lemon juice   1 teaspoon fresh lemon zest, grated finely

¼ cup fresh cilantro, chopped

> In a pan, add water wheat berries and pinch of salt over high heat and bring to a boil. Reduce the heat to low and simmer, covered for about 60-90 minutes or until tender enough. Drain well and transfer into a large bowl.

> Meanwhile, preheat the grill to medium-high heat. Grease the grill grate.

> Coat the eggplant slices with 2 tablespoons of oil.

> Grill the eggplant slices and tomatoes for about 8-10 minutes, flipping occasionally. Remove the vegetables from grill.

> Transfer the tomatoes onto a cutting board. Peel off the skin of tomatoes and chop them.

> Transfer the eggplants, tomatoes and Serrano chile into the bowl with berries and mix. With mortar and pestle, pound the garlic cloves with a pinch of salt into a paste. Stir in 2 tablespoons of oil, spices, lemon juice and zest.

> Heat a small non-stick frying pan over medium-low heat and sauté garlic mixture for about 2 minutes. Add remaining oil and stir vigorously until well combined.

> Transfer the garlic mixture and cilantro into the bowl with berry salad and toss to coat well. Keep aide to cool completely.

> Divide salad into 4 airtight containers and refrigerate for 1 day.

Servings **4**   Per Serving**:**   *Calories* **386**   *Protein* **10.6g**   *Carbohydrates* **51g**   *Fat* **18.8g**

Soba Noodles Salad

For Salad:
    4-ounce soba noodles

    1 red bell pepper, seeded and sliced thinly

    1 green bell pepper, seeded and sliced thinly

    1 cup cooked edamame, shelled

    2 large carrots, peeled and shredded

    6 scallions, sliced thinly

    ½ cup crunchy rice noodles

For Dressing:
    2 teaspoons peanut butter   4 teaspoons soy sauce

    4 teaspoons rice vinegar   4 teaspoons chili paste

    ¼ cup extra-virgin olive oil

    1 tablespoon black sesame seeds

> Cook the noodles according to package's directions.

> Meanwhile, for dressing: in a bowl, add all ingredients except oil and sesame seeds and beat until well combined. Slowly, add oil, beating continuously until smooth. Gently, stir in sesame seeds.

> In the bottom of 4 large mason jars, divide the dressing evenly. Divide the salad ingredients in the layers of soba noodles, followed by bell pepper, edamame, carrot, scallion and rice noodles.

> Cover each jar with the lid tightly and refrigerate for about 1 day. Shake the jars well just before serving.

Servings **4**   Per Serving: Calories **414**   Protein **15.6g**   Carbohydrates **46.9g**   Fat **20.7g**

Rice & Mango Salad

For Rice: 3 cups water   1½ cups brown rice

For Dressing: 2/3 cup fresh orange juice   2 tablespoons balsamic vinegar

2 tablespoons vegetable oil   2 tablespoons honey

2 teaspoons orange zest, grated freshly   2 tablespoons honey

Salt, to taste

For Salad: 2 large oranges, peeled, seeded and chopped

3 cups fresh spinach, torn   1/3 cup red onion, sliced

> In a large pan, add water and rice over high heat and bring to a boil. Reduce the heat to low and simmer, covered for about 45-60 minutes or until all the liquid is absorbed. Transfer the rice into a large bowl.

> Meanwhile, in another medium bowl, add all dressing ingredients and beat until well combined. Pour the dressing over hot rice and stir to combine.

> In a third bowl, mix together all salad ingredients.

> Divide rice and salad into 4 airtight containers and refrigerate for 1-2 days.

Servings **4**   Per Serving: Calories **455**   Protein **7.3g**   Carbohydrates **88.7g**   Fat **9g**

Rice & Tofu Salad

For Salad:
- 1 (12-ounce) package tofu, drained and sliced
- 1½ cups steamed rice
- ½ of cucumber, peeled, seeded and chopped
- ½ of head romaine lettuce, torn

For Dressing:
- 3 scallions, chopped
- 2 tablespoons black sesame seeds, toasted
- 2 tablespoons soy sauce
- ½ teaspoon sesame oil, toasted
- Drop of hot pepper sauce
- 1 teaspoon white sugar
- 1¼ teaspoons chile pepper powder

> In a large serving bowl, add all salad ingredients and mix. In another bowl, add all dressing ingredients and beat until well combined. Pour dressing over salad and gently toss to coat well.

> Divide salad into 4 airtight containers and refrigerate for 1 day.

Servings **4**   Per Serving**:**   *Calories* **365**   *Protein* **213.8g**   *Carbohydrates* **62.6g**   *Fat* **6.9g**

Curried Chicken Soup

1½ pounds chicken breasts, cut into 1½-inch pieces

2 cups chicken broth

2 (12-ounces) cans coconut milk

1 red bell pepper, seeded, sliced

2 tablespoons red curry paste

2 tablespoons brown sugar

2 tablespoons fish sauce

2 tablespoons peanut butter

1 onion, thinly sliced

1 tablespoon fresh ginger, minced

1 cup frozen peas, thawed

1 tablespoon fresh lime juice

> In a slow cooker, add chicken breast pieces, chicken broth, coconut milk, bell pepper, red curry paste, brown sugar, fish sauce, peanut butter, onion and ginger. Set the cooker on Low and cook, covered for about 4½ hours.

> Uncovered and stir in peas. Set the cooker on Low and cook, covered for about ½ hour.

> Uncover and keep aside to cool completely.

> Transfer soup into 6 individual meal prep containers. Cover and store in refrigerator for up to 5 days. Reheat soup before serving.

Servings **6**   Per Serving: Calories **592**   Protein **40.5g**   Carbohydrates **19.5g**   Fat **40.5g**

Creamy Chicken Soup

1 tablespoon extra-virgin olive oil

1 large sweet onion, chopped

4 garlic cloves, minced

2 cups carrots, peeled and sliced

1 red bell pepper, seeded and chopped

1¼ pounds boneless, skinless chicken breasts

1½ teaspoons dried thyme

Salt and freshly ground black pepper, to taste

9 cups chicken broth

1 (8.8-ounce) package three cheese tortellini

½ cup fresh baby spinach

¼ cup heavy cream

2 tablespoons fresh parsley, chopped

> In a large pan, heat oil over medium heat and sauté onion and garlic for about 3 minutes. Add carrot and bell pepper and sauté for about 3 minutes. Add chicken breasts, thyme, salt and black pepper and bring to a boil. Reduce the heat and simmer for about 15 minutes. With a slotted spoon, transfer chicken breasts onto a cutting board. Cut chicken into bite sized pieces.

> Increase heat to medium and stir in cheese tortellini. Add chopped chicken and cook for about 10-15 minutes, stirring occasionally. Remove from heat and immediately, stir in spinach, heavy cream and parsley.

> Remove from heat and keep aside to cool slightly.

> Transfer soup into 6 individual meal prep containers. Cover and store in refrigerator for up to 5 days. Reheat soup before serving.

Servings **6**   Per Serving: Calories **440**   Protein **42g**   Carbohydrates **28g**   Fat **16.9g**

Chicken & Potato Soup

4 bacon slices, chopped   1 large onion, chopped   3 garlic cloves, minced

3 pounds russet potatoes, peeled and sliced thinly

1½ pounds boneless skinless chicken breasts   2 cups carrots, peeled and sliced

2 cup celery stalks, sliced   8 cups chicken broth   1 teaspoon dried thyme

1/3 cup fresh parsley, chopped   Salt and freshly ground black pepper, to taste

> Heat a skillet over medium heat and cook bacon until browned. Add onions and garlic and sauté for about 3-4 minutes. Transfer onions mixture into a slow cooker.

> Place chicken breast over onions, followed by potatoes, carrots, celery, chicken broth, thyme, salt and black pepper. Set the slow cooker on High and cook, covered for about 8-12 hours, stirring occasionally.

> Transfer chicken breast onto a cutting board. Cut into bite sized pieces. With an immerse blender, puree the soup. Stir in chicken and remove from heat. Keep aside to cool completely.

> Transfer soup into 8 individual meal prep containers. Cover and store in refrigerator for up to 5 days. Reheat soup before serving.

Servings **8**   Per Serving: *Calories* **422**   *Protein* **38.4g**   *Carbohydrates* **33.7g**   *Fat* **14g**

Chicken & Sweet Potato Soup

1 tablespoon olive oil

½ cup onion, chopped

1 carrot, peeled and chopped

2 celery stalks, chopped

2 garlic cloves, minced

1 tablespoon fresh oregano, chopped

1 tablespoon fresh parsley, chopped

1 teaspoon fresh ginger, minced

6 cups chicken broth

1 cup sweet potato, peeled and spiralized

1 cup cooked chicken, shredded

Salt and freshly ground black pepper, to taste

2 tablespoons fresh lemon juice

> In a large soup pan, heat oil over medium heat and sauté onion, carrot and celery for about 3-4 minutes. Add garlic, ginger, oregano and parsley and sauté for about 1 minute. Add broth and bring to a boil over high heat. Reduce the heat to low and simmer for about 15-20 minutes. Add sweet potato and cooked chicken and simmer for about 8-10 minutes. Stir in salt, black pepper and lemon juice and remove from heat. Keep aside to cool slightly.

> Transfer soup into 4 individual meal prep containers. Cover and store in refrigerator for up to 5 days. Reheat soup before serving.

Servings | **4** | Per Serving**:** | Calories | **208** | Protein | **19.1g** | Carbohydrates | **16.6g** | Fat | **7g**

Chicken & Veggie Soup

3 tablespoons olive oil

2 cups yellow onion, chopped

1 cup celery, sliced thinly

4 garlic cloves, minced

2-3 cups green cabbage, sliced thinly

8 cups chicken broth

2 (15-ounce) cans cannellini beans, drained and rinsed

3-4 cups cooked chicken, shredded

1 tablespoon dried oregano

1 tablespoon dried oregano

Salt and freshly ground black pepper, to taste

2 cups fresh kale, trimmed and chopped

1 cup zucchini, chopped

2 tablespoons fresh lemon juice

> In a large pan, heat oil over medium-high heat and sauté onion, celery and garlic for about 5-6 minutes. Add cabbage and sauté for about 3 minutes, stirring occasionally. Add the garlic and sauté for about 1-2 minutes. broth, beans, shredded chicken, dried herbs, salt and black pepper and bring to a boil. Boil for about 5 minutes. Stir in kale, zucchini and lemon juice and bring to a boil. Cook for about 1-2 minutes.

> Remove from heat and keep aside to cool completely.

> Transfer soup into 12 individual meal prep containers. Cover and store in refrigerator for up to 5 days. Reheat soup before serving.

Servings **12**   Per Serving: *Calories* **368**   *Protein* **31.1g**   *Carbohydrates* **48.3g**   *Fat* **6.2g**

Chicken & Noodles Soup

2 tablespoons olive oil

1 large yellow onion, chopped

Salt, to taste

2 garlic cloves, minced

3 large carrots, peeled and chopped

3 celery stalks, chopped

4 skinless, boneless chicken breasts

4 cups chicken broth

2½-ounce fresh spinach

> In a large pan, heat oil over medium-high heat and sauté onion and a little salt for about 3-5 minutes. add garlic and sauté for about 1 minute. Add carrots and celery and cook for about 4-5 minutes. Add chicken breasts and broth and bring to a boil. Reduce heat to low and simmer for about 25 minutes.

> Uncover the pan and transfer chicken breasts onto a cutting board. Cut chicken breasts into bite size pieces. Add chicken and spinach into pan and cook for about 3-4 minutes.

> Remove from heat and keep aside to cool completely.

> Transfer soup into 4 individual meal prep containers. Cover and store in refrigerator for up to 5 days. Reheat soup before serving.

Servings **4**   Per Serving**:**   *Calories* **359**   *Protein* **39.2g**   *Carbohydrates* **11.2g**   *Fat* **16.9g**

Chicken & Quinoa Soup

- 2 skinless, boneless chicken breasts, cubed
- ½ cup quinoa, rinsed
- ¼ cup dried yellow split peas
- 6-8 carrots, chopped
- 6-8 celery stalks, chopped
- 1 large onion, chopped
- 2 garlic cloves, minced
- 6 cups chicken broth
- 2 cups water
- 1 tablespoon Cajun spice seasoning
- 1 teaspoon smoked paprika
- Salt and freshly ground black pepper, to taste

> In a slow cooker, place all ingredients. Set the slow cooker on Low and cook, covered for about 6 hours. Serve in a serving bowl.

> Uncover and keep aside to cool completely.

> Transfer soup into 6 individual meal prep containers. Cover and store in refrigerator for up to 5 days. Reheat soup before serving.

Servings **6** Per Serving**:** Calories **267** Protein **26.3g** Carbohydrates **24.3g** Fat **6.7g**

Turkey & Spinach Soup

4 teaspoons extra-virgin olive oil

½ teaspoon fresh ginger, minced

6-ounce ground turkey

¼ cup canned water chestnuts, sliced

1 tablespoon hot chili pepper

5 cups fresh spinach, torn

½ cup scallion, chopped

2 garlic cloves, minced

1 cup bean sprouts

3 cups chicken broth

2 tablespoons soy sauce

> In a medium soup pan, heat 1 teaspoon of oil over medium heat and sauté scallion, ginger and garlic for about 1 minute. Add ground turkey and cook for about 4-5 minutes. Drain off excess fat from pan. Add bean sprouts, water chestnuts, chicken broth, hot chili pepper and soy sauce and bring to a boil over medium-high heat. Reduce the heat to low and simmer for about 15 minutes. Stir in spinach and cook for about 3-4 minutes more.

> Remove from heat and keep aside to cool completely.

> Transfer soup into 3 individual meal prep containers. Cover and store in refrigerator for up to 5 days. Reheat soup before serving.

Servings **3**   Per Serving: Calories **251**   Protein **25.6g**   Carbohydrates **9.1g**   Fat **14.4g**

Beef & Mushroom Soup

2 tablespoons olive oil

2 garlic cloves, minced

8-ounce New York strip steak, cubed

1 cup white onion, chopped

1 teaspoon dried thyme, crushed

1½ cups shiitake mushrooms, sliced

3 cups bone broth

1 tablespoon soy sauce

½ cup fresh cilantro leaves, chopped

1 tablespoon scallion (green part), chopped

1 tablespoon fresh lemon juice

> In a soup pan, heat 1 tablespoon of oil over medium heat and sauté garlic for about 1 minute. Add beef and cook for about 4-5 minutes or until browned. Transfer the beef into a bowl.

In the same pan, heat remaining oil over medium heat and sauté onion for about 4-5 minutes. Add thyme and mushrooms and cook for about 3-4 minutes. Add broth and bring to a boil. Reduce the heat to low. Stir in soy sauce and beef and simmer for about 10 minutes. Stir in cilantro and lemon juice and remove from heat. Keep aside to cool completely.

> Transfer soup into 4 individual meal prep containers. Cover and store in refrigerator for up to 5 days. Reheat soup before serving.

Servings **4**   Per Serving: *Calories* **249**   *Protein* **25.8g**   *Carbohydrates* **12.1g**   *Fat* **11.1g**

Beef & Barley Soup

2 pounds beef chuck roast, cubed

1 (8-ounces) can tomato sauce

½ onion, chopped finely

5 cups beef broth

¾ cup uncooked pearl barley

> In a slow cooker, place all ingredients. Set the cooker on Low and cook, covered for about 5 hours.

> Uncover and keep aside to cool completely.

> Transfer soup into 6 individual meal prep containers. Cover and store in refrigerator for up to 5 days. Reheat soup before serving.

Servings | **6**   Per Serving**:**   *Calories* | **818**   *Protein* | **56g**   *Carbohydrates* | **27.7g**   *Fat* | **52.3g**

Pork & Sweet Potato Soup

1 tablespoon olive oil

1 teaspoon fresh ginger, minced

2 garlic cloves, minced

½ teaspoon dried thyme, crushed

½ teaspoon ground cumin

¼ teaspoon ground coriander

½ teaspoon red pepper flakes, crushed

1 pound lean ground pork

Salt and freshly ground black pepper, to taste

4 cups chicken broth

1 medium sweet potato, peeled and spiralized

4 cups fresh spinach, torn

1 cup scallion, chopped

> In a large soup pan, heat oil over medium heat and sauté ginger, garlic, thyme and spices for about 1 minute. Add beef, salt and black pepper and cook for about 9-10 minutes, stirring and breaking with a spoon. Add broth and bring to a boil. Reduce the heat to low and simmer for about 8-10 minutes. Add sweet potato and simmer for about 5 minutes. Add spinach and scallion and simmer for about 3- 4 minutes more. Season with required salt and black pepper and remove from heat. Keep aside to cool completely.

> Transfer soup into 4 individual meal prep containers. Cover and store in refrigerator for up to 5 days. Reheat soup before serving.

Servings **4**   Per Serving**:**   *Calories* **345**   *Protein* **26.3g**   *Carbohydrates* **10.9g**   *Fat* **22.3g**

Sausage & Beans Soup

1 tablespoon olive oil   1 pound ground sausage

1 yellow onion, chopped finely   2 garlic cloves, minced

4 cups fresh kale, trimmed and chopped   6 cups chicken broth

2 (14-ounce) cans white beans, rinsed

Salt and freshly ground black pepper, to taste

> In a large non-stick skillet, heat olive oil over medium heat and cook ground sausage until browned. Add onion and garlic and cook for about 2-4 minutes. Slowly, add kale, 1 cup at a time and cook until wilted.

> Transfer the cooked mixture to the slow cooker. Add broth, white beans, salt and black pepper. Set the slow cooker on High and cook, covered for about 3 hours.

> Uncover and keep aside to cool completely.

> Transfer soup into 8 individual meal prep containers. Cover and store in refrigerator for up to 5 days. Reheat soup before serving.

Servings **8**   Per Serving**:**   *Calories* **590**   *Protein* **39g**   *Carbohydrates* **65.5g**   *Fat* **19.7g**

Salmon & Cabbage Soup

- 2 tablespoons olive oil
- 1 shallot, chopped
- 2 small garlic cloves, minced
- 1 jalapeño pepper, chopped
- 1 head cabbage, chopped
- 2 small red bell pepper, seeded and chopped finely
- 5 cups vegetable broth
- 2 (4-ounce) salmon boneless fillets, cubed
- ¼ cup fresh cilantro, minced
- 2 tablespoons fresh lemon juice
- Freshly ground black pepper, to taste

> In a large soup pan, heat oil over medium heat and sauté shallot and garlic for 2-3 minutes. Add cabbage and bell peppers and sauté for about 3-4 minutes. Add broth and bring to a boil over high heat. Reduce the heat to medium-low and simmer for about 10 minutes. Add salmon and cook for about 5-6 minutes. Stir in the cilantro, lemon juice and black pepper and cook for about 1-2 minutes.

> Remove from heat and keep aside to cool completely.

> Transfer soup into 4 individual meal prep containers. Cover and store in refrigerator for up to 5 days. Reheat soup before serving.

Servings **4**   Per Serving: Calories **255**   Protein **20.3g**   Carbohydrates **17.7g**   Fat **12.6g**

Shrimp & Bell Pepper Soup

2 tablespoons olive oil
1 pound fresh medium shrimp, peeled and deveined
2 teaspoons red curry paste
2 garlic cloves, minced
1 teaspoon fresh ginger, minced
1 green bell peppers, seeded and chopped
1 red bell peppers, seeded and chopped
6 cups fish broth
1¾ cups unsweetened coconut milk
2 tablespoons fresh lime juice
Salt and freshly ground black pepper, to taste
½ cup scallion, chopped

> In a large soup pan, heat oil over medium-high heat and cook shrimp for about 2-3 minutes. With a slotted spoon transfer the shrimp into a large plate.

> In the same pan, add curry paste, garlic and ginger and sauté for about 1 minute. Add bell peppers and cook for about 3-4 minutes. Add broth and coconut milk and bring to a boil on high heat. Reduce the heat to low and simmer for about 8-10 minutes. Stir in lime juice, shrimp and scallion and cook for about 2 minutes.

> Remove from heat and keep aside to cool completely.

> Transfer soup into 8 individual meal prep containers. Cover and store in refrigerator for up to 5 days. Reheat soup before serving.

Servings | **8**   Per Serving: *Calories* | **369**   *Protein* | **189.3g**   *Carbohydrates* | **10.3g**   *Fat* | **29.2g**

Mussels & Corn Soup

4 ears sweetcorn   1 tablespoon olive oil   2 celery stalks, chopped

1 small white onion, chopped   1 fresh red chili, seeded and chopped finely

1 sweet potato, peeled and chopped   3 cups chicken broth

1 cup fresh mussels, scrubbed and debearded

> Peel the husk from corn ears and with a sharp knife cut off the kernels. Keep aside.

> In a pan, heat oil on medium-low heat and sauté celery and onion for about 5 minutes. Add sweet potato, sweet corn and broth and bring to a boil. Reduce the heat to low and simmer for about 10-15 minutes. Remove from heat and keep aside to cool slightly.

> In a blender, add soup in batches and pulse until smooth. Return the soup in the pan and stir in mussels. Bring to a boil cook for about 3-5 minutes. Season with salt and black pepper and remove from heat. Keep aside to cool completely.

> Transfer soup into 4 individual meal prep containers. Cover and store in refrigerator for up to 5 days. Reheat soup before serving.

Servings **4**   Per Serving: *Calories* **257**   *Protein* **13.9g**   *Carbohydrates* **38.8g**   *Fat* **7.3g**

Barley & Beans Soup

2 tablespoons coconut oil

1 white onion, chopped

2 celery stalks, chopped

1 large carrot, peeled and chopped

2 garlic cloves, minced

2 tablespoons fresh rosemary, chopped

4 cups fresh tomatoes, chopped finely

4 cups vegetable broth

1 cup pearl barley

2 cups cooked white beans

2 tablespoons fresh lemon juice

> In a large soup pan, melt coconut oil over medium heat and sauté onion, celery and carrot for about 4-5 minutes. Add garlic and rosemary and sauté for about 1 minute. Add tomatoes and cook for 3-4 minutes, crushing with back of spoon. Add broth and barley and bring to a boil. Reduce the heat to low and simmer, covered for about 20-25 minutes. Stir in beans and lemon juice and simmer for 5 minutes more.

> Remove from heat. Keep aside to cool completely.

> Transfer soup into 4 individual meal prep containers. Cover and store in refrigerator for up to 5 days. Reheat soup before serving.

Servings **4**   Per Serving: *Calories* **669**   *Protein* **35.7g**   *Carbohydrates* **113.8g**   *Fat* **10.3g**

Beans & Greens Soup

1 tablespoon olive oil	1 medium onion, chopped
2 celery stalks, chopped	2 medium carrots, peeled and chopped
2 garlic cloves, minced	2 tablespoons fresh thyme, minced
2 cups fresh tomatoes, chopped finely	3 cups fresh spinach, chopped
3 cups fresh kale, trimmed and chopped	2 cups cooked white beans
8 cups vegetable broth	Salt and freshly ground black pepper, to taste

> In a large soup pan, heat oil over medium heat and sauté onion, celery and carrot for about 5-6 minutes. Add garlic and thyme and sauté for about 1 minute. Add tomatoes and cook for about 2 to 3 minutes, crushing with the back of spoon. Add remaining all ingredients and bring to a boil over high heat. Reduce the heat to low and simmer, covered for about 20-30 minutes.

> Remove from heat. Keep aside to cool completely.

> Transfer soup into 8 individual meal prep containers. Cover and store in refrigerator for up to 5 days. Reheat soup before serving.

Servings **8**   Per Serving**:**   *Calories* **260**   *Protein* **18.5g**   *Carbohydrates* **39.7g**   *Fat* **3.8g**

Beans & Broccoli Soup

¾ pound broccoli head, chopped

1 onion, chopped

1 jalapeño pepper, seeded and chopped

1½ cups cooked cannellini beans

Salt and freshly ground black pepper, to taste

1 tablespoon olive oil

2 garlic cloves, minced

2½ cups vegetable broth

> In a pan of boiling water, add the broccoli and cook for about 3-4 minutes. Drain well.

> In a large soup pan, heat oil on medium heat and sauté onion for about 5 minutes. Add garlic and jalapeño pepper and sauté for about 1 minute. Add broth and beans and bring to a boil.

> Remove from heat and keep aside to cool slightly. In a blender, add soup and broccoli and pulse in batches until smooth. Return the soup in the pan and cook for about 3-4 minutes. Season with salt and black pepper and remove from heat. Keep aside to cool completely.

> Transfer soup into 4 individual meal prep containers. Cover and store in refrigerator for up to 5 days. Reheat soup before serving.

Servings | **4**   Per Serving: *Calories* | **326**   *Protein* | **22.1g**   *Carbohydrates* | **50.7g**   *Fat* | **5.3g**

Two-Beans Soup

1 cup cooked red kidney beans

1 cup cooked white kidney beans

2 tablespoons fresh rosemary, chopped

Salt and freshly ground black pepper, to taste

2 cups hot vegetable broth

1 teaspoon olive oil

> In a high-speed blender, add all ingredients except oil and pulse until smooth.

> Transfer soup into 4 individual meal prep containers. Cover and store in refrigerator for up to 5 days. Reheat soup before serving.

Servings **4**   Per Serving: Calories **343**   Protein **23.7g**   Carbohydrates **57.3g**   Fat **0.8g**

Lentil & Veggie Soup

1 tablespoon olive oil   4 scallions, chopped   3½ cups tomatoes, chopped

6 cups vegetable broth   ½ cup brown lentils

2 sweet potatoes, peeled and cut into ½-inch pieces

4 cups fresh kale, trimmed and chopped   1 tablespoon fresh thyme, chopped

Salt and freshly ground black pepper, to taste

> In a large soup pan, heat oil over medium heat and sauté scallions for about 3-4 minutes. Add tomatoes and cook for 3-4 minutes, crushing with the back of spoon. Add broth and bring to a boil. Add lentils, sweet potato, kale and thyme and again bring to a boil. Reduce the heat to low and simmer, covered for about 25-30 minutes or until desired doneness. Season with salt and black pepper and remove from heat.

> With an immense blender, puree the soup. Keep aside to cool completely.

> Transfer soup into 6 individual meal prep containers. Cover and store in refrigerator for up to 5 days. Reheat soup before serving.

Servings | **6**   Per Serving**:**   *Calories* | **219**   *Protein* | **12.2g**   *Carbohydrates* | **34.2g**   *Fat* | **4.2g**

Quinoa & Carrot Soup

For Soup:　　5 cups unsweetened almond milk, divided

　　　　　　5½ cups carrots, peeled and chopped

　　　　　　1 teaspoon ground cinnamon　　1 teaspoon ground ginger

　　　　　　1 teaspoon sweet paprika　　½ teaspoon ground cumin

　　　　　　Salt and freshly ground black pepper, to taste

For Quinoa:　2 cups water　　½ cup quinoa　　1½ tablespoons olive oil

　　　　　　Salt, to taste

> For soup in a large soup pan, add 3 cups of almond milk and remaining ingredients and bring to a boil over high heat. Reduce the heat to medium-low and simmer for about 15-20 minutes. Remove from heat and let it cool slightly.

> In a blender, add soup mixture in batches and pulse until smooth. Transfer the soup and remaining almond milk in pan and cook for about 4-5 minutes.

> Meanwhile in another pan of salted boiling water, add quinoa ad cook for about 8-10 minutes. Drain well and transfer into a bowl.

> In a non-stick skillet, heat oil over medium heat and cook quinoa and salt for about 5-7 minutes, stirring continuously.

Add quinoa into carrot soup ant stir to combine. Keep aside to cool completely.

> Transfer soup into 8 individual meal prep containers. Cover and store in refrigerator for up to 5 days. Reheat soup before serving.

Servings **8**　Per Serving:　*Calories* **120**　*Protein* **2.8g**　*Carbohydrates* **16.1g**　*Fat* **5.5g**

Lentil & Quinoa Soup

½ cup red quinoa   1 cup dry lentils   ½ cup mushrooms, sliced

½ cup carrots, peeled and chopped   1 cup celery stalk, chopped

1 tablespoon ground ginger   1 tablespoon ground cumin

½ tablespoon chili powder   1 teaspoon red pepper flakes, crushed

4 cups water

> In a large soup pan, mix together all ingredients over high heat and bring to a boil. Reduce the heat to medium-low and simmer, covered for about 45-60 minutes or until lentil becomes tender.

> Remove from heat and keep aside to cool completely.

> Transfer soup into 4 individual meal prep containers. Cover and store in refrigerator for up to 5 days. Reheat soup before serving.

Servings **4**   Per Serving: *Calories* **251**   *Protein* **15.5g**   *Carbohydrates* **42.6g**   *Fat* **2g**

Root Veggies Soup

2 tablespoons olive oil   1 onion, chopped   2 garlic cloves, minced

¼ teaspoon dried thyme, crushed   ¼ teaspoon ground cumin

1/8 teaspoon red pepper flakes, crushed   1/8 teaspoon smoked paprika

1 cup carrot, peeled and chopped   2 sweet potatoes, peeled and chopped

1 turnip, peeled and chopped   1 parsnip, peeled and chopped

2½ cups vegetable broth   Salt and freshly ground black pepper, to taste

> In a large soup pan, heat oil over medium heat and sauté onion for about 4-5 minutes. Add garlic, thyme and spices and sauté for about 1 minute. Add carrots, sweet potatoes and turnip and cook for about 10 minutes. Add broth and bring to a boil. Reduce the heat to low and simmer for about 15-20 minutes.

> Remove from heat and keep aside to cool slightly. In a blender, add soup in batches and pulse until smooth. Season with salt and black pepper and keep aside to cool completely.

> Transfer soup into 3 individual meal prep containers. Cover and store in refrigerator for up to 5 days. Reheat soup before serving.

Servings **3**   Per Serving**:**   *Calories* **309**   *Protein* **7.4g**   *Carbohydrates* **47.2g**   *Fat* **10.9g**

Chicken & Chickpeas Stew

6 pounds skinless, boneless chicken thighs, trimmed

Salt and freshly ground black pepper, to taste

¼ cup extra-virgin olive oil

3 large yellow onions, sliced thinly

8 garlic cloves, crushed

3 red chiles, stemmed

1 tablespoon ground turmeric

2 teaspoon ground coriander

2 teaspoons ground cumin

4 teaspoons fresh lemon zest, grated finely

½ cup fresh lemon juice, divided

4 cups chicken broth

2 cups small green olives, pitted

2 cups canned chickpeas, rinsed and drained

> Season the chicken thighs with salt and black pepper evenly.

> In a large pan, heat oil over medium-high heat and cook chicken thighs in 4 batches for about 3 minutes per side. Transfer the chicken into a bowl and keep aside.

> In the same pan, add onion over medium and sauté for about 5-6 minutes. Add garlic, red chiles and spices and sauté for about 1 minute. Add lemon zest, 1/3 cup of the lemon juice and broth and bring to a boil. Reduce the heat to medium-low and simmer, covered for about 30 minutes. Add cooked chicken, olives and chickpeas and remove from heat. Increase the heat to medium-high and cook for about 6-8 minutes, stirring occasionally. Stir in remaining lemon juice, salt and black pepper and remove from heat. Keep aside to cool completely.

> Transfer stew into 12 individual meal prep containers. Cover and store in refrigerator for up to 5 days. Reheat before serving.

Servings | **12**　　Per Serving:　　Calories | **309**　　Protein | **7.4g**　　Carbohydrates | **47.2g**　　Fat | **10.9g**

Beef & Pumpkin Stew

1 pound beef stew meat, trimmed and cubed

Salt and freshly ground black pepper, to taste

2 tablespoons olive oil, divided

2 medium carrots, peeled and chopped

2 celery stalks, chopped

1 medium onion, chopped

1 cup pumpkin, peeled and cubed

3 cups fresh tomatoes, chopped finely

4 cups water

1 cup frozen peas, thawed

> Season the beef with a little salt and black pepper evenly.

In a large pan, heat 1 tablespoon of oil over medium heat and sear beef for about 4-5 minutes. Transfer the beef in a large bowl and keep aside.

> In the same pan, heat remaining oil over medium heat and sauté carrot, celery and onion for about 5 minutes Add pumpkin and tomatoes and sauté for about 5 minutes. Add broth and beef and bring to a boil over high heat. Reduce the heat to low and simmer, covered for about 1 hour. Uncover and simmer for about 35 minutes. Stir in peas, salt and black pepper and simmer for 15 minutes more.

> Remove from heat and keep aside to cool completely.

> Transfer stew into 5 individual meal prep containers. Cover and store in refrigerator for up to 5 days. Reheat before serving.

Servings **5**   Per Serving: *Calories* **296**   *Protein* **31.1g**   *Carbohydrates* **17g**   *Fat* **11.8g**

Beef & Squash Stew

1½ tablespoons coconut oil, divided

2-3 pounds stew meat, trimmed and cubed into 1½-inch size

1 onion, chopped   ½ teaspoon fresh ginger, minced

5 garlic cloves, minced   2 cups bone broth

1 butternut squash, peeled and cubed   ¼ teaspoon ground cinnamon

2 pears, cored and chopped

> In a large heavy bottomed pan, heat 1 tablespoon of oil over medium-high heat and sear beef for about 8-10 minutes or until browned completely. With a slotted spoon, transfer the beef into a bowl.

> In the same pan, add onion over medium and sauté for about 5 minutes. Add ginger and garlic and sauté for about 2 minutes. Add cooked beef and broth and bring to a boil. Reduce the heat to low and simmer, covered for about 15 minutes. Stir in squash, cinnamon and salt and simmer, covered for about 15 minutes. Stir in pears and simmer, covered for about 30 minutes.

> Remove from heat and keep aside to cool completely.

> Transfer stew into 6 individual meal prep containers. Cover and store in refrigerator for up to 5 days. Reheat before serving.

Servings | **6**   Per Serving**:**   Calories | **669**   Protein | **66.9g**   Carbohydrates | **37.2g**   Fat | **28.2g**

Lamb Stew

1 teaspoon ground cumin　　1 teaspoon ground coriander

½ teaspoon cayenne pepper　　½ teaspoon ground cinnamon

2 tablespoons olive oil　　3 pounds lamb stew meat, trimmed and cubed

Salt and freshly ground black pepper, to taste　　1 onion, chopped

2 garlic cloves, minced　　2¼ cups chicken broth

2 cups tomatoes, chopped finely

1 medium head cauliflower, cut into 1-inch florets

> Preheat the oven to 300 degrees F.

> In a small bowl, mix together spices and keep aside.

> In a large ovenproof pan, heat oil over medium heat and cook lamb with a little salt and black pepper for about 10 minutes or until browned from all sides. Transfer the lamb into a bowl.

> In the same pan, add onion and sauté for about 3-4 minutes. Add garlic and spice mixture and sauté for about 1 minute. Add cooked lamb, broth and tomatoes and bring to a gentle boil. Immediately, cover the pan and transfer into oven.

> Bake for about 1½ hours. Remove from oven and stir in cauliflower. Bake for about 30 minutes more or until cauliflower is done completely.

> Remove from oven and keep aside to cool completely.

> Transfer stew into 8 individual meal prep containers. Cover and store in refrigerator for up to 5 days. Reheat before serving.

Servings **8**　Per Serving:　Calories **409**　Protein **52.6g**　Carbohydrates **11.3g**　Fat **16.7g**

Haddock Stew

2 large Yukon Gold potatoes, sliced into ¼-inch size

1 tablespoon olive oil

½ teaspoon fresh ginger, chopped finely

1 (16-ounce) can whole tomatoes, crushed

½ cup water

1 cup clam juice

¼ teaspoon red pepper flakes, crushed

Salt, to taste

1½ pounds boneless haddock, cut into 2-inch pieces

> Arrange a steamer basket in a large pan of water and bring to a boil. Place the potatoes in steamer basket and cook, covered for about 8 minutes.

> Meanwhile in a pan, heat oil over medium heat and sauté ginger for about 1 minute. Add tomatoes and cook, stirring continuously for about 2 minutes. Add water, clam juice, red pepper flakes and bring to a boil. Simmer for about 5 minutes, stirring occasionally. Gently, stir in haddock pieces and simmer, covered for about 5 minutes or until desired doneness.

> Remove from heat and keep aside to cool completely.

> Divide haddock into 4 individual meal prep containers and top with stew. Cover and store in refrigerator for up to 5 days. Reheat before serving.

Servings **4**   Per Serving: Calories **295**   Protein **35.5g**   Carbohydrates **26.4g**   Fat **5.2g**

Seafood Stew

- 2 tablespoons coconut oil
- ½ cup onion, chopped finely
- 2 garlic cloves, minced
- 1 Serrano pepper, chopped
- 1 teaspoon smoked paprika
- 4 cups fresh tomatoes, chopped
- 4 cups chicken broth
- 1 pound salmon fillets, cubed
- ½ pound shrimp, peeled and deveined
- ½ pound fresh bay scallops, rinsed and dried
- 2 tablespoons fresh lime juice
- ¼ cup fresh basil, chopped
- ¼ cup fresh parsley, chopped
- Salt and freshly ground black pepper, to taste

> In a large soup pan, melt coconut oil over medium-high heat and sauté onion for about 5-6 minutes. Add garlic, Serrano pepper and smoked paprika and sauté for about 1 minute. Add tomatoes and broth and bring to a gentle boil. Reduce heat to o medium and simmer for about 5 minutes. Add salmon and simmer for about 3-4 minutes. Stir in remaining seafood and cook for about 4-5 minutes. Stir in lemon juice, basil, parsley, salt and black pepper and remove from heat. Keep aside to cool completely.

> Transfer stew into 6 individual meal prep containers. Cover and store in refrigerator for up to 5 days. Reheat before serving.

Servings **6**   Per Serving**:**   *Calories* **272**   *Protein* **34.3g**   *Carbohydrates* **8.5g**   *Fat* **11.3g**

Chickpeas & Squash Stew

1 tablespoon olive oil

1 medium sweet onion, chopped

½ teaspoons fresh ginger, grated

2 garlic cloves, minced

½ tablespoon coconut sugar

¼ teaspoon ground cumin

¾ teaspoon ground cinnamon

1-2 teaspoons red chili flakes, crushed

3½ cups butternut squash, peeled and chopped

Salt and freshly ground black pepper, to taste

1½ cups water, divided

¼ cup creamy natural almond butter

1½ cups cooked chickpeas

3 cups fresh kale, trimmed and chopped

½ cup raw almonds, chopped

> In a large soup pan, heat oil over medium heat and cook onion, covered for about 5 minutes, stirring occasionally. Stir in ginger, garlic, coconut sugar and spices and sauté for about 1 minute. Add squash and stir to combine well. Add 1¼ cups of water, salt and black pepper and bring to a boil. Reduce the heat to low.

> In a bowl, mix together remaining water and peanut butter. Add peanut butter mixture in pan and stir to combine. Simmer, covered for about 20 minutes. Stir in chickpeas, kale and almonds and simmer for about 10 minutes more.

> Remove from heat. Keep aside to cool completely.

> Transfer stew into 6 individual meal prep containers. Cover and store in refrigerator for up to 5 days. Reheat before serving.

Servings **6** Per Serving: Calories **383** Protein **16.2g** Carbohydrates **51.2g** Fat **14.9g**

Mixed Veggie Stew

2 tablespoons coconut oil

1 large sweet onion, chopped

1 medium parsnips, peeled and chopped

3 tablespoons tomato paste

2 large garlic cloves, minced

½ teaspoon ground cinnamon

½ teaspoon ground ginger

1 teaspoon ground cumin

¼ teaspoon cayenne pepper

2 medium carrots, peeled and chopped

2 medium purple potatoes, peeled and chopped

2 medium sweet potatoes, peeled and chopped

4 cups vegetable broth

2 tablespoons fresh lemon juice

2 cups fresh kale, kale, trimmed and chopped

> In a large soup pan, melt coconut oil over medium-high heat and sauté onion for about 5 minutes. Add parsnip and sauté for about 3 minutes. Stir in tomato paste, garlic and spices and sauté for about 2 minutes. Stir in carrots, potatoes and sweet potatoes and broth and bring to a boil. Reduce the heat to medium-low and simmer, covered for about 20 minutes. Stir in lemon juice and kale and simmer for about 4-5 minutes

> Keep aside to cool completely.

> Transfer stew into 8 individual meal prep containers. Cover and store in refrigerator for up to 5 days. Reheat before serving.

Servings **8**   Per Serving: *Calories* **171**   *Protein* **5.3g**   *Carbohydrates* **28.6g**   *Fat* **4.4g**

Veggies & Rice Stew

2½ cups water

3 carrots, peeled and chopped

1 parsnip, peeled and chopped

1 onion, chopped

½ teaspoon cayenne pepper

Salt and freshly ground black pepper, to taste

3 potatoes, scrubbed and chopped

1 turnip, peeled and chopped

¼ cup uncooked rice

1 teaspoon ground cumin

> In a large pan, add water and bring to a boil over medium-high heat. Add remaining ingredients and again bring to a boil. Reduce the heat to medium and cook for about 30 minutes.

> Remove from heat and keep aside to cool completely.

> Transfer stew into 4 individual meal prep containers. Cover and store in refrigerator for up to 5 days. Reheat before serving.

Servings **4** Per Serving: Calories **214** Protein **4.9g** Carbohydrates **48.7g** Fat **0.5g**

Bee Curry

2 tablespoons olive oil, divided

1 pound boneless beef, trimmed and cut into thin strips

Salt and freshly ground black pepper, to taste

1 white onion, chopped

1 red bell pepper, seeded and chopped

1 garlic clove, minced

1 teaspoon fresh ginger, minced

1 teaspoon curry powder

1 cup coconut milk

2 medium zucchinis, spiralized

2 medium yellow squash, spiralized

2 tablespoons fresh lime juice

> In a large pan, heat 1 tablespoon of oil over medium heat and cook beef and with salt and black pepper for about 4-5 minutes or until browned. Transfer the beef into a bowl.

> In the same pan, heat remaining oil over medium heat and sauté onion and bell pepper for about 3-4 minutes. Add garlic and curry powder and sauté for 1 minute, slowly, add coconut milk and bring to a boil. Stir in beef and cook for 4-5 minutes. Add zucchini and squash and cook for about 4-5 minutes. Stir in lime juice, salt and black pepper and remove from heat. Keep aside to cool completely.

> Transfer curry into 4 individual meal prep containers. Cover and store in refrigerator for up to 5 days. Reheat before serving.

Servings | **4**   Per Serving**:**   Calories | **459**   Protein | **36.2g**   Carbohydrates | **14.3g**   Fat | **28.8g**

Salmon Curry

¼ cup coconut oil, divided

½ of red onion, chopped finely

3 garlic cloves, minced

1 teaspoon curry powder

½ teaspoon ground turmeric

Salt, to taste

¼ cup fresh cilantro, chopped

½ teaspoon mustard seeds

1 teaspoon fresh ginger, minced

2 green chiles, seeded and chopped

1 teaspoon ground cumin

1½ cups full-fat coconut milk

4 (6-ounce) salmon fillets

> In a large pan, heat 2 tablespoons of oil over medium heat and sauté mustard seeds for about 30 seconds. Add onion and sauté for about 3-4 minutes. Add ginger and garlic and sauté for about 30 seconds. Add green chiles, curry powder, cumin and turmeric and sauté for 4-5 minutes. Stir in coconut milk and salt and bring to a boil. Reduce the heat to low and simmer for about 15 minutes.

> Meanwhile, in a large skillet, heat remaining oil over medium heat and cook salmon fillets for about 2-3 minutes, flipping once in the middle way.

> Transfer the fish into pan of simmering sauce and simmer for 5 minutes. Stir in cilantro and remove from heat. Keep aside to cool completely.

> Transfer curry into 4 individual meal prep containers. Cover and store in refrigerator for up to 5 days. Reheat before serving.

Servings **4**   Per Serving: *Calories* **563**   *Protein* **35.5g**   *Carbohydrates* **7.7g**   *Fat* **45.8g**

Mushroom & Corn Curry

- 2 cup tomatoes, chopped
- 1 teaspoon fresh ginger, chopped
- 2 tablespoons canola oil
- ¼ teaspoon ground coriander
- ¼ teaspoon red chili powder
- 1½ cups fresh button mushrooms, sliced
- 1¼ cups water
- 1 Serrano pepper, chopped
- ¼ cup cashews
- ½ teaspoon cumin seeds
- ¼ teaspoon ground turmeric
- 1½ cups fresh shiitake mushrooms, sliced
- 1 cup frozen corn kernels
- ¼ cup coconut milk

> In a food processor, add tomatoes, Serrano, ginger and cashews and pulse until a smooth paste forms.

> In a pan, heat oil on medium heat and sauté cumin seeds for about 1 minute. Add spices and sauté for about 1 minute. Add tomato paste and cook for about 5 minutes. Stir in mushrooms, corn, water and coconut milk and cook for about 10-12 minutes, stirring occasionally.

> Remove from heat. Keep aside to cool completely.

> Transfer curry into 3 individual meal prep containers. Cover and store in refrigerator for up to 5 days. Reheat before serving.

Servings **3**   Per Serving: Calories **290**   Protein **6g**   Carbohydrates **27.4g**   Fat **20.2g**

Lentil & Apple Curry

- 8 cups water
- ½ teaspoon ground turmeric
- 1 cup brown lentils
- 1 cup red lentil
- 1 tablespoon vegetable oil
- 1 large white onion, chopped
- 3 garlic cloves, minced
- 2 tomatoes, seeded and chopped
- 1½ tablespoons curry powder
- ¼ teaspoon ground cloves
- 2 teaspoons ground cumin
- 2 carrots, peeled and chopped
- 2 potatoes, scrubbed and chopped
- 2 cups pumpkin, peeled, seeded and cubed into 1-inch size
- 1 granny smith apple, cored and chopped
- 2 cups fresh spinach, chopped
- Salt and freshly ground black pepper, to taste

> In a large pan, add water, turmeric and lentils and bring to a boil over high heat. Reduce the heat to medium-low and simmer, covered for about 45 minutes. Drain the lentils, reserving 2½ cups of cooking liquid.

> In a large pan, heat oil over medium heat and sauté onion for about 2-3 minutes. Add garlic and sauté for about 1 minute. Add tomatoes and cook for about 5 minutes. Stir in curry powder and spices and cook for about 1 minute. Add carrots, potatoes, pumpkin, cooked lentils and reserved cooking liquid and bring to a gentle boil. Reduce the heat to medium-low and simmer, covered for about 35-45 minutes or until desired doneness of vegetables. Stir in apple and spinach and simmer for about 15 minutes.

> Remove from heat. Keep aside to cool completely.

> Transfer curry into 6 individual meal prep containers. Cover and store in refrigerator for up to 5 days. Reheat before serving.

Servings **6**   Per Serving: Calories **315**   Protein **17.3g**   Carbohydrates **63g**   Fat **3.6g**

Cashew Chicken

For Sauce: 3 garlic cloves, minced   1 tablespoon fresh ginger, grated

2 tablespoons tomato paste

3 tablespoons coconut palm sugar   ¼ cup coconut vinegar

1/3 cup soy sauce

½ teaspoon red pepper flakes, crushed

For Chicken: 2 pounds skinless, boneless chicken thighs, cut into bite-sized pieces

2 tablespoons arrowroot powder

Salt and freshly ground black pepper, to taste

2 tablespoons olive oil

1 green bell peppers, seeded and chopped

1 red bell peppers, seeded and chopped

½ cups raw cashews   2 large scallions, chopped

> In a bowl, add all sauce ingredients and beat until well combined. Keep aside.

> In another large bowl, add chicken, arrowroot powder, salt and black pepper and toss to coat well. Keep aside for at least 10 minutes.

> In a large skillet, heat oil over medium-high heat and sauté bell peppers for about 2-3 minutes. Transfer the bell pepper into a bowl.

> In the same skillet, add chicken mixture and stir fry for about 6-8 minutes. Slowly, add sauce, stirring continuously. Stir in cashews and cooked bell peppers and bring to a gentle simmer. Reduce the heat to medium-low and simmer for about 3-5 minutes or until desired thickness. Stir in scallion and remove from heat. Keep aside to cool completely.

> Transfer chicken mixture into 8 individual meal prep containers. Cover and store in refrigerator for up to 5 days. Reheat before serving.

Servings **8**   Per Serving: *Calories* **268**   *Protein* **27.9g**   *Carbohydrates* **13.9g**   *Fat* **11.7g**

Chicken & Veggies

2 medium skinless, boneless chicken breasts, cut into ½-inch pieces

1 medium zucchini, chopped

1 cup fresh broccoli florets

1 small red onion, chopped

2 garlic cloves, minced

1 teaspoon Italian seasoning

1 teaspoon Italian seasoning

½ teaspoon paprika

Salt and freshly ground black pepper, to taste

2 tablespoons olive oil

4 cups cooked rice

> Preheat the oven to 450 degrees F. Line a large baking dish with a piece of foil.

> In a large bowl, add all ingredients except rice and toss to coat well. Transfer the chicken mixture onto prepared baking dish in a single layer.

> Bake for about 15-20 minutes or until the chicken is tender.

> Remove from oven and keep aside to cool completely.

> Divide rice and chicken mixture into 4 individual meal prep containers. Cover and store in refrigerator for up to 5 days. Reheat before serving.

Servings **4** Per Serving: *Calories* **906** *Protein* **12.9g** *Carbohydrates* **153.5g** *Fat* **12.9g**

Chicken with Cauliflower Rice

For Chicken: 2 tablespoons olive oil

1 pound boneless, skinless chicken breast

Salt and freshly ground black pepper, to taste

¼ cup fresh lime juice   1/3 cup fresh cilantro, chopped

2 teaspoons garlic, minced   ½ teaspoon honey

For Cauliflower Rice: 2 tablespoons olive oil   3 cups cauliflower ric

2 teaspoons garlic powder   1 teaspoon ground cumin

Salt, to taste   ½ cup black beans

¼ cup red onion, sliced thinly

> For Chicken in a large skillet, heat oil over medium heat over medium heat and cook chicken for about 5-8 minutes per side. Remove from heat and keep aside to cool slightly. Cut chicken into slices.

> In a large bowl, add remaining ingredients and mix well. Add chicken slices and toss to coat well.

> For Cauliflower rice: in a large skillet, heat oil over medium heat and cook cauliflower rice and spices for about 5 minutes. Stir in black beans and sauté for about 2 minutes. stir in red onion and remove from heat.

> Keep chicken and cauliflower rice mixture aside to cool completely.

> Divide chicken and cauliflower rice mixture into 4 individual meal prep containers. Cover and store in refrigerator for up to 5 days. Reheat before serving.

Servings | 4   Per Serving: Calories | 371   Protein | 37.3g   Carbohydrates | 22.9g   Fat | 17.4g

Stuffed Chicken Cutlets

6 chicken breast culets

Salt and freshly ground black pepper, to taste

9 smoked ham slices

10 Swiss cheese slices

½ cup unsalted butter, melted

1½ cups plain panko breadcrumbs

1 tablespoon dried parsley flakes, crushed

> Preheat the oven to 375 degrees F. Grease 8 mason jars.

> Place a large plastic wrap onto a large smooth surface. Arrange chicken cutlets onto plastic wrap so they overlap each other a little. Cover the cutlets with another large plastic wrap. With a meat mallet, pound the cutlets into a large and thin chicken sheet. Remove the upper plastic wrap and sprinkle with salt and black pepper evenly. Place ham slices over chicken sheet, followed by cheese slices evenly. With plastic wraps, roll the chicken sheet into a log shape. With a sharp knife, cut the log into 8 (1½-1¾-inch thick) slices. Carefully, remove the plastic wrap from each slice.

> Divide the chicken slices into prepared mason jars.

> In a bowl, mix together butter, breadcrumbs, parsley, salt and black pepper. Place the breadcrumbs mixture over each chicken slice evenly.

> Arrange the jars in a rimmed baking sheet and bake for about 20 minutes. Remove from oven and cover each jar with foil pieces. Bake for about 15 minutes. Uncover the jars and bake for about 5 minutes more.

> Remove from oven and keep aside to cool completely.

> Cover each jar with the lid tightly and refrigerate for about 1 day. Reheat slightly before serving.

Servings | 6   Per Serving: Calories | **747**   Protein | **41.3g**   Carbohydrates | **49.6g**   Fat | **44.4g**

Mini Chicken Pies

2 packages frozen pie crusts

1/3 cup onion, chopped

Salt and freshly ground black pepper, to taste

1¾ cups chicken broth

1 package mixed frozen vegetables (peas and broccoli)

3 cups cooked chicken, shredded

1/3 cup butter

1/3 cup all-purpose flour

½ cup milk

> Preheat the oven to **425 degrees F.**

> Cut each of the pie crust into quarters. Arrange 1 piece in each of 8 Mason jars to cover the jar completely.

> In a large skillet, melt butter over medium heat and sauté onion for about 2 minutes. Add flour, salt and black pepper and until well combined. Slowly, add the broth and milk, stirring continuously. Cook until mixture becomes thick, stirring continuously. Stir in the frozen vegetables and stir fry for about 2-3 minutes. Stir in chicken and remove from heat.

> Divide the chicken mixture in prepared jars evenly Place the remaining crust quarters over the filling in each jar. Cut the dough to adjust the size. With a knife, make the vents in top.

> Arrange the jars onto a rimmed baking sheet and bake for about 15 minutes. Cover the jars with a foil paper and bake for 15-20 minutes more.

> Remove from oven and keep aside to cool completely.

> Cover each jar with the lid tightly and refrigerate for about 1-2 days. Reheat slightly before serving.

Servings | **8**   Per Serving: Calories | **275**   Protein | **19.4g**   Carbohydrates | **14.9g**   Fat | **15.2g**

Beef in Milky Sauce

1 pound lean ground beef

¼ cup onion, chopped

1 teaspoon beef bouillon powder

¼ cup flour

¼ teaspoon onion powder

¼ teaspoon garlic powder

¼ teaspoon cayenne pepper

Salt and freshly ground black pepper, to taste

2¼ cups milk

½ teaspoon Worcestershire sauce

> Heat a large nonstick skillet over medium heat and cook beef for about 4-5 minutes. Add onion and cook for about 4-5 minutes. Stir in beef bouillon powder, flour, onion powder, garlic powder, cayenne pepper, salt and black pepper and cook for about 5 minutes or until flour is absorbed completely, stirring continuously. Add milk and Worcestershire sauce and bring to a gentle simmer. Cook for about 5-10 minutes, stirring continuously or until mixture becomes thick.

> Remove from oven and keep aside to cool completely.

> Divide beef mixture into 4 individual meal prep containers. Cover and store in refrigerator for up to 5 days. Reheat before serving.

Servings **4**   Per Serving: *Calories* **312**   *Protein* **39.9g**   *Carbohydrates* **13.7g**   *Fat* **10g**

Chicken Sausage with Veggies

1 tablespoon olive oil

6 Italian chicken sausages, sliced

1 cup snow peas

1 large red bell pepper, seeded and sliced thinly

1 large orange bell pepper, seeded and sliced thinly

1 teaspoon garlic powder

Salt and freshly ground black pepper, to taste

> In a large skillet, heat oil over medium-high heat and cook sausage for about 8-10 minutes. Transfer the sausage slices into a large bowl and keep aside.

> In the same skillet, add snow peas, bell peppers and garlic powder and sauté for about 3-5 minutes. Stir in sausage, salt and black pepper and remove from heat.

> Remove from heat and keep aside to cool completely.

> In 4 containers, divide sausage mixture evenly and refrigerate for about 1 day. Reheat before serving.

Servings **4** Per Serving: Calories **182** Protein **9.8g** Carbohydrates **11.9g** Fat **10.9g**

Pork with Pineapple

2 tablespoons coconut oil   1½ pound pork tenderloin, cut into bite-sized pieces

1 onion, chopped   2 garlic cloves, minced   1 teaspoon fresh ginger, minced

20-ounce fresh pineapple, cut into chunks

1 large red bell pepper, seeded and chopped   ¼ cup fresh pineapple juice

¼ cup soy sauce   Salt and freshly ground black pepper, to taste

> In a large skillet, heat oil over medium heat and cook pork for about 4-5 minutes. Transfer the pork into a large bowl and keep aside.

> In the same skillet, add onion and sauté for about 4-5 minutes. Add garlic and ginger and sauté for about 1 minute. Add pineapple and bell pepper and cook for about 3-4 minutes. Stir in pineapple juice, soy sauce, salt, black pepper and cooked pork and cook for about 4-5 minutes.

> Remove from heat and keep aside to cool completely.

> In 6 containers, divide sausage mixture evenly and refrigerate for about 1 day. Reheat before serving.

Servings **6**   Per Serving: *Calories* **276**   *Protein* **31.4g**   *Carbohydrates* **18.3g**   *Fat* **8.7g**

Lamb with Couscous

¾ cup couscous   ¾ cup boiling water   ¼ cup fresh cilantro, chopped

1 tablespoon olive oil   5-ounce lamb leg steak, cubed into ¾-inch size

1 medium zucchini, sliced thinly   1 medium red onion, cut into wedges

1 teaspoon ground cumin   1 teaspoon ground coriander

¼ teaspoon red pepper flakes, crushed   Salt, to taste

> In a large bowl, add couscous and boiling water and stir to combine, Cover and keep aside for about 5 minutes. Add cilantro and with a fork, fluff completely.

> Meanwhile, in a large skillet, heat oil over high heat and stir fry lamb for about 2-3 minutes. Add zucchini and onion and stir fry for about 2 minutes. Stir in spices and stir fry for about 1 minute Add couscous and stir fry for about 2 minutes.

> Remove from heat and keep aside to cool completely.

> In 2 containers, divide lamb mixture evenly and refrigerate for about 1 day. Reheat before serving.

Servings **2**   Per Serving: *Calories* **479**   *Protein* **30.2g**   *Carbohydrates* **59.3g**   *Fat* **13.1g**

Veggies Combo

3 tablespoon canola oil, divided

1 medium green bell pepper, seeded and chopped finely

1 medium onion, chopped finely   1 garlic clove, minced

8-ounce fresh mushrooms, sliced

½ of (16-ounce) package frozen okra, thawed, trimmed and sliced

1 (14½-ounce) can diced tomatoes with liquid   1 (6-ounce) can tomato paste

1 teaspoon dried thyme, crushed   ½ teaspoon cayenne pepper

¼ teaspoon red pepper flakes, crushed

Salt and freshly ground black pepper, to taste   2 tablespoons all-purpose flour

> In a large pan, heat 1 tablespoon of oil over medium heat and sauté bell pepper, onion and garlic for about 4-5 minutes. Stir in mushrooms, okra, tomatoes, tomato paste, bay leaves, thyme and spices and cook for about 40 minutes, stirring occasionally.

> In a frying pan, heat remaining oil over medium heat. Slow, add flour, stirring continuously. Cook for about 3-5 minutes or until a roux is formed, for about 40 minutes.

> Add the roux in gumbo mixture, stirring continuously. Cook for about 5-10 minutes, , stirring occasionally.

> Remove from heat and keep aside to cool completely.

> In 6 containers, divide gumbo evenly and refrigerate for about 1 day. Reheat before serving.

Servings **6**   Per Serving: Calories **146**   Protein **4.5g**   Carbohydrates **17.6g**   Fat **7.6g**

Mini Veggies Pies

For Topping:
- 3 medium Yukon Gold potatoes, peeled and cubed
- 3 cups fresh kale, trimmed and chopped
- 1 scallion, chopped
- 1½ tablespoons butter
- ¾ cup milk
- 1/8 teaspoon freshly ground nutmeg
- Salt, to taste

For Filling:
- 1½ tablespoons olive oil, divided
- 14-ounces vegetarian sausage, crumbled
- 2 medium carrots, peeled and chopped finely
- 1 medium onion, chopped
- 3 celery stalks, chopped
- 1 cup cabbage, chopped
- 2 garlic cloves, minced
- Salt and freshly ground black pepper, to taste
- 2 tablespoons flour
- ½ cup vegetable broth
- ½ cup Guinness
- 2 teaspoons Worcestershire sauce
- 1 cup frozen peas, thawed
- ¼ cup fresh parsley, chopped

> Preheat the oven to 400 degrees F.

> For topping in a pan of water, add potatoes and bring to a boil over high heat. Reduce the heat to low and simmer for about 25 minutes. Drain the potatoes and return in the same pan and with a potato masher, mash the potatoes and cover the pan.

> Meanwhile, in another pan, add remaining topping ingredients except cheese and bring to a gentle simmer. Simmer, covered for about 10-12 minutes, stirring occasionally.

> Transfer the kale mixture in the pan of potatoes and stir to combine. Cover the pan and remove from heat.

> For filling: in skillet, heat 1 tablespoon of oil over medium-high heat and cook sausage and cook until browned completely. Transfer the sausage into a plate.

> In the same skillet, heat the remaining oil and cook onion, carrot, celery, cabbage, garlic, salt and black pepper for about 10-12 minutes. Add flour and stir until well coated with vegetables. Add broth, Guinness and Worcestershire sauce and cook until mixture becomes thick, stirring continuously. Add sausage, peas and parsley and cook until heated completely.

> In 6 mason jars, divide filling mixture and top with the topping mixture evenly. Arrange the jars onto a rimmed baking sheet and bake for about 20 minutes. Now, switch the oven settings to broiler. Broil for about 1-3 minutes or until top becomes golden brown.

> Remove from oven and keep aside to cool completely.

> Cover each jar with the lid tightly and refrigerate for about 1-2 days. Reheat slightly before serving.

Servings | **6**   Per Serving: *Calories* | **336**   *Protein* | **9.8g**   *Carbohydrates* | **36.8g**   *Fat* | **11.8g**

Mixed Grains Combo

¾ cup amaranth   1 cup quinoa   ¼ cup wild rice   4 cups water

2 teaspoons ground cumin   ½ teaspoon paprika   Salt, to taste

1 cup canned chickpeas, drained and rinsed   ½ cup raisins

2 medium carrots, peeled and grated   1 garlic clove, minced

Salt and freshly ground black pepper, to taste

> In a large pan, mix together amaranth, quinoa, wild rice, water and spices over medium-high heat and bring to a boil. Reduce the heat to medium-low and simmer, covered for about 20-25 minutes. Stir in remaining ingredients and remove from heat. Serve immediately.

> Remove from heat and keep aside to cool completely.

> In 6 containers, divide gumbo evenly and refrigerate for about 1 day. Reheat before serving.

Servings **6**   Per Serving: Calories **389**   Protein **15.7g**   Carbohydrates **71.7g**   Fat **5.6g**

Final Words

Thank you again for picking up this cookbook! I hope it was able to help you to find a wide variety of simple and delicious sounding recipes that you can't wait to try for yourself.

Finally, if you enjoyed this book, then I'd like to ask you for a favor, would you be kind enough to leave a review for this book? It'd be greatly appreciated!